2025
18天攻克
医学考博

英语核心词 第③版

环球卓越医学考博命题研究中心 / 组编

梁莉娟　赵牧童 / 编著

U0378775

机械工业出版社
CHINA MACHINE PRESS

本书作为已有良好市场声誉的卓越医学考博英语应试教材的单本，由全国知名医学博士英语统考培训机构"环球卓越"策划，联手医学博士资深辅导专家，在对近10年真题词频统计的基础上，结合大纲要求，对词频为3以上的单词进行精选、精讲，并针对医学博士考生时间紧、战线长、记忆压力大等现实情况，将学习任务分解成18天，化整为零，去粗取精，内容精炼。同时本书配套音频朗读，加之口袋大小的设计，携带便捷，考生随时随地可记忆单词。

图书在版编目（CIP）数据

18天攻克医学考博英语核心词／环球卓越医学考博命题研究中心组编；梁莉娟，赵牧童编著. -- 3版. 北京：机械工业出版社，2024. 8. -- （卓越医学考博英语应试教材）. -- ISBN 978 - 7 - 111 - 76626 - 1

Ⅰ. R

中国国家版本馆 CIP 数据核字第 2024JT9215 号

机械工业出版社（北京市百万庄大街22号　邮政编码100037）

策划编辑：孙铁军	责任编辑：孙铁军　苏筛琴
责任校对：夏晓琳	责任印制：单爱军

保定市中画美凯印刷有限公司印刷

2024 年 9 月第 3 版第 1 次印刷
105mm×148mm · 4.5 印张 · 170 千字
标准书号：ISBN 978 - 7 - 111 - 76626 - 1

定价：32.80 元

电话服务　　　　　　　　　　网络服务
客服电话：010 - 88361066　　机 工 官 网：www.cmpbook.com
　　　　　010 - 88379833　　机 工 官 博：weibo. com/cmp1952
　　　　　010 - 68326294　　金 书 网：www. golden-book. com
封底无防伪标均为盗版　　机工教育服务网：www.cmpedu.com

丛书序

这是一套由全国知名医学博士英语统考培训机构"环球卓越"（优路教育旗下品牌）策划，联手医学博士英语资深辅导专家，为众多志在考取医学博士的考生量身定制的应试辅导用书。国家医学考试中心于2019年底修订了考试大纲，对全国医学博士外语统一考试的题型及各部分分值进行了局部调整。新大纲仍然设置了听力对话、听力短文、词语用法、完形填空、阅读理解和书面表达6种题型，但调整了具体命题形式，其中听力部分变化最大。"15个短对话+1个长对话+2个短文"的经典组合成为历史，从2020年开始，"5个短对话+5个小短文"的搭配将在很长一段时间内成为考生要面对的题型。考试时间为3个小时（含播放录音及收发卷时间）。

考纲的变化并未改变对考生能力的考查方向，因此为了帮助广大考生在较短的时间内系统备考，在听、说、读、写4个方面得到强化训练，全面提高英语应用和交际能力，顺利通过考试，本套"卓越医学考博英语应试教材"仍然是广大考生朋友们很好的选择。本丛书紧密结合最近几年卫生部组织的医学博士英语统一考试命题情况，针对最新考试大纲进行了修订，并针对新题型编写了大量针对性练习。本丛书包含《全国医学博士英语统考词汇巧战通关》《全国医学博士英语统考综合应试教程》《全国医学博士英语统考实战演练》三本传统综合分册，《医学考博阅读理解高分全解》《医学考博英语听力28天训练计划》两本专项分册，以及《18天攻克医学考博英语核心词》的单词小分册。传统分册从基础到综合再到真题实战，从模块详解到全套试题，高屋建瓴，逐步推进。阅读专项分册对分值较高的阅读理解进行字、词、句、语篇的详解和训练，从技术（语言知识）到技巧（做题方法），精讲多练。听力专项分册则根据听力训练的规律和考试考查目标，按天设置训练内容，分解目标，逐步达成最终目标。

本丛书的特点如下：

一、紧贴考试，实用性强

策划编写本丛书的作者常年在教学一线授课，从基础英语到医博考前辅导，积累了大量的应试辅导实战经验。丛书内容是他们多年辅导经验的提炼和结晶，实用性非常强，专为医学考博考生定制，是目前市面上较全面、系统的医学考博英语应试教材。

二、紧扣大纲，直击真题

本丛书紧扣最新大纲，体例设置与大纲保持一致；各部分考点紧密结合最新历年真题，还原真实考场环境，命题思路分析透彻，重点突出，讲解精确；各部分内容严格控制在大纲规定的范围之内，让考生准确把握考试的重点、难点及命题趋势。

三、内容精练，讲练结合

传统分册《全国医学博士英语统考词汇巧战通关》《全国医学博士英语统考综合应试教程》和《全国医学博士英语统考实战演练》简单精练，通过突破词汇基础关、学习各种题型应试方法以及在高质量实战中历练，考生可在有限的时间内进行全面复习，把握重点，比较系统地完成考前准备。阅读分册《医学考博阅读理解高分全解》则是根据考生的具体情况，分模块予以详解，提升基础，总结技巧，各个击破。听力专项《医学考博英语听力28天训练计划》则专练听力，循序渐进，按天分配学习任务，力争高分。核心词汇专项《18天攻克医学考博英语核心词》在使用词频软件完整统计近十年全套真题的基础上，将该统计结果和大纲词汇进行比较，最后确定出记忆任务的内容和安排。按天设置，不断重复。

四、超值服务，锦上添花

本丛书附带赠送精品服务，由优路教育为每位购书读者提供专业的服务和强大的技术支持。具体为：

1.《医学考博英语听力28天训练计划》附赠内容：优路教育"2025年医学考博（统考）《英语听力28天

训练计划》图书赠课英语（20节）"网络视频课程。使用方法：刮开书籍封底的兑换码，扫描书籍封底二维码关注【优路医学考试】微信公众账号后，点击【兑换课程】-【点击这里兑换课程】的链接，输入兑换码，输入姓名手机号，将自动跳转至您的课程页，开始观看课程。后续看课路径：关注【优路医学考试】服务号，在底部菜单栏【我要学习】-【我的课程】查看课程。（可通过扫描文末二维码，关注后兑换课程）

2.《18天攻克医学考博英语核心词》附赠内容：优路教育"2025年医学考博（统考）《18天攻克医学考博英语核心词》图书赠课英语（20节）"网络视频课程。使用方法：刮开书籍封底的兑换码，扫描书籍封底二维码关注【优路医学考试】微信公众账号后，点击【兑换课程】-【点击这里兑换课程】的链接，输入兑换码，输入姓名手机号，将自动跳转至您的课程页，开始观看课程。后续看课路径：关注【优路医学考试】服务号，在底部菜单栏【我要学习】-【我的课程】查看课程。（可通过扫描文末二维码，关注后兑换课程）

3.《全国医学博士英语统考实战演练》附赠内容：优路教育"2025年医学考博（统考）《实战演练》图书赠课英语（10节）"网络视频课程。使用方法：刮开书籍封底的兑换码，扫描书籍封底二维码关注【优路医学考试】微信公众账号后，点击【兑换课程】-【点击这里兑换课程】的链接，输入兑换码，输入姓名手机号，将自动跳转至您的课程页，开始观看课程。后续看课路径：关注【优路医学考试】服务号，在底部菜单栏【我要学习】－【我的课程】查看课程。（可通过扫描文末二维码，关注后兑换课程）

4.《全国医学博士英语统考综合应试教程》附赠内容：优路教育"2025年医学考博（统考）《综合应试教程》图书赠课英语（10节）"网络视频课程。使用方法：刮开书籍封底的兑换码，扫描书籍封底二维码关注【优路医学考试】微信公众账号后，点击【兑换课程】－【点击这里兑换课程】的链接，输入兑换码，输入姓名手机号，将自动跳转至您的课程页，开始观看课程。后续看课路径：关注【优路医学考试】服务号，在底部菜单栏【我要学习】－【我的课程】查看课程。（可通过扫描文末二维码，关注后兑换课程）

5.《全国医学博士英语统考综词汇巧战通关》附赠内容：优路教育"2025年医学考博（统考）《词汇巧战通关》图书赠课【学习卡】英语（10节）"网络视频课程。使用方法：刮开书籍封底的兑换码，扫描书籍封底二维码关注【优路医学考试】微信公众账号后，点击【兑换课程】－【点击这里兑换课程】的链接，输入兑换码，输入姓名手机号，将自动跳转至您的课程页，开始观看课程。后续看课路径：关注【优路医学考试】服务号，在底部菜单栏【我要学习】－【我的课程】查看课程。（可通过扫描文末二维码，关注后兑换课程）

6.《医学考博阅读理解高分全解》附赠内容：优路教育"2025年医学考博（统考）《阅读理解高分全解》图

书赠课【学习卡】英语（8节）"网络视频课程。使用方法：刮开书籍封底的兑换码，扫描书籍封底二维码关注【优路医学考试】微信公众账号后，点击【兑换课程】－【点击这里兑换课程】的链接，输入兑换码，输入姓名手机号，将自动跳转至您的课程页，开始观看课程。后续看课路径：关注【优路医学考试】服务号，在底部菜单栏【我要学习】－【我的课程】查看课程。（可通过扫描文末二维码，关注后兑换课程）

优路教育技术支持及服务热线 400－8835－981，可以帮您解决兑换及观看课程中的技术问题。您也可以登录优路教育网站 www.youlu.com，在"医学博士英语"栏目下获取更多的学习资料和资讯。

编　者

2024 年 4 月于北京

扫码关注后兑换课程

前　言

医学博士入学英语考试的词汇复习是个大难题。"词汇词汇，必须要背"，道理都懂，可考生总在不甘心地四处探寻：背什么？怎么背？作为一个研究英语考试多年的一线英语老师来讲，我们着实也无法说出更多天花乱坠的奇妙方法，无法装出手里握着天下无二的记忆妙方的样子。读者们都是准博士了，英语水平先放一边不论，逻辑思维能力和归纳总结水平一定已经炉火纯青了，那么一定能判断，背单词无论是顺序记忆、乱序记忆，抑或词根词缀记忆、谐音记忆，都脱离不了两个字：重复。但重复是要有内涵的。重复两遍5000个词，或许和重复10遍1000个词所用时间相差无几，但结果一定是大相径庭。前者大约能对500个词"有印象"，而后者能将500个词熟稔于心。因此，绝大多数考生都认同且追求把有限的时间用于尽可能少的内容的记忆。

这就是编写《18天攻克医学考博英语核心词》的思路：浓缩记忆内容，设置重复场景。尽可能地创造"10（遍）×1000（词）"的机会。记忆内容可不能乱减，必须有权威指引和科学基础。研究再三，我们采取了"从真题出发，向大纲进攻"的路径：使用词频软件完整统计近十年的全套真题，再将该统计结果和大纲词汇进行比较，最后确定出记忆任务的层次和要求，先搞定真题，再填补和大纲的差距。而对于"重复"的机会，我们则设置成"3 周×7 天－3 天（休息检测日）"的模式，即 18 天、每天不到 100 个单词的单日任务，目的就在于使考生有不断重复的可能性。

从统计结果中不难发现，词频超过 10 次的，往往是初中词汇（甚至小学词汇），比如排名最前的 the、to、of 等（后附详细统计结果），这些单词的记忆要求层次为"唤醒"，因此，我们在附录一放置了词频统计表，附录二放置了小词大用，侧重超高额的虚词。建议考生打印，不断检测、扫描、唤醒，换言之，此部分单词不需要背诵，而是筛查。

按常理，备考应该手握大纲，循序渐进，从头背起。但通过研究真题发现，医学博士入学英语考试的词汇范围，在实际命题中并非严格以大纲为蓝本，考生认为不重要的，不一定是命题人不考的，比如 antidioxide。换言之，四六级的考试经验，未见得完全适用于医博英语考试，毕竟有"医学"这个限定词。基于这种现实情况，我们将词频 3～10 之间的词汇与大纲进行对照，删掉基础词汇，补进真题词汇，最后形成了这本书的记忆主体。

18 天的记忆任务原则上是按字母排序规划的，但为了减少"顺序记忆"中的心理压力（从 A 到 Z，遥遥无期），我们进行了字母组合，比如 A＋Z，B＋Q

等，本部分采用的是【联想】【搭配】【导学】【例句】的体例，提供不同的记忆路径，以便记忆时能事半功倍。【联想】则是"联想词"和"派生词"，这样做可以让考生开阔视野，举一反三，成串记忆。【搭配】则是该词的特殊用法、习惯搭配等。【导学】重在辨析近义词。【例句】大多从历年真题中挑选经典句子来讲解词汇，并配有译文。

如前所述，附录中放入词频统计和小词大用的结果全文，大家可自行排序，有参照地复习。如果考生朋友想要更详细的工具书，则可移步《全国医学博士英语统考词汇巧战通关》，那里应有尽有。

本书同时配套词汇朗读音频和讲解视频，不方便用阅读的方式复习的时候，耳朵也是可以随时打开接受英语的"刺激"的，这有助于维持自己复习的状态，将碎片化时间利用到极致。

感谢广大考生和众多老师在编写过程中提供的建议和帮助。由于时间仓促，书中难免有错误及遗漏之处，欢迎批评指正。

编者

2024 年 7 月 12 日

目 录

Day *1*

abandon [əˈbændən]　　　　　　*vt.* 放弃，抛弃，离弃

【联想】 give up doing sth. / quit doing sth. 放弃做某事

【导学】 abandon 后接动名词，如：abandon doing sth. 放弃做某事。

【例句】 But even if some disasters meant that the vault was abandoned, the permanently frozen soil would keep the seeds alive.

【译文】 但是，即使某些灾难意味着储藏室被遗弃了，永远冰冻的土地也会使种子保持活力。

ability [əˈbiliti]　　　　　　*n.* 能力，智能；才能，才干

【搭配】 of great/exceptional ability 能力卓越
　　　　of high/low/average ability 能力高/低/一般
　　　　to the best of one's ability 尽其所能

【联想】 able 能的—unable 不能的
　　　　ability 能力—inability 无能
　　　　enable 使能够—disable 使无能，使伤残

【例句】 Adolescents simply lack the ability to make smart decisions consistently.

【译文】 青少年只是缺乏始终如一地做出明智决定的能力。

1

abnormal [æb'nɔːməl]　　　　　　　　*a.* 不正常的

【联想】abnormally *ad.* 不正常地

【例句】The so-called Mad Cow Disease is caused by abnormal proteins coming into contact with neurons in the brain.

【译文】所谓"疯牛病"，是异常蛋白质侵入脑神经原引起的。

abolish [ə'bɔliʃ]　　　　　　　　　　*vt.* 废除，取消

【例句】The first step is to abolish the existing system.

【译文】首先要废除现行体制。

abroad [ə'brɔːd]　　　　　　　*ad.* 国外，海外；传开

【搭配】at home and abroad 国内外

absent ['æbsənt]　　*a.* 缺席的；缺乏的；漫不经心的

【搭配】be absent from 缺席

【联想】absence *n.* 缺席，缺乏

【例句】I need to be absent from class on Friday morning because I have a doctor's appointment.

【译文】周五早晨的课我要缺席了，因为我要看医生。

absolute ['æbsəluːt]　　　　　*a.* 绝对的；完全的

【例句】Sometimes we buy a magazine with absolutely

no purpose other than to pass time.

【译文】有时我们买杂志是完全没有目的的，仅仅是为了打发时间。

absorb [əb'sɔːb]　　　　*vt.* 吸收；吸引，使专心

【搭配】be absorbed in 全神贯注于

【联想】absorption *n.* 吸收

【例句】That makes it harder for your body to absorb calcium in the presence of caffeine, thus increasing your rate of bone loss.

【译文】那使得你的身体因咖啡因的存在而更难吸收钙，从而增加你骨质流失的速度。

abuse [ə'bjuːs]　　　　*n.* 滥用；虐待；辱骂
　　　　　[ə'bjuːz]　　　　*vt.* 滥用；虐待；辱骂

【搭配】abuse one's authority 滥用职权

【联想】abuser *n.* 滥用者；abusive *a.* 滥用的

【例句】The abuse of alcohol and drugs is also a common factor.

【译文】酗酒和吸毒是常见的因素。

academic [ˌækə'demik]　　　　*a.* 学院的；学术的

【联想】academia *n.* 学术界；academics *n.* 学术

【例句】The effective work of maintaining discipline is usually performed by students who advise the academic authorities.

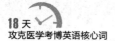

【译文】有效地维持纪律通常是由学生来做的，这些学生负责给学校的领导提建议。

accelerate [ək'seləreit]　v. 加快；加速；(使) 加速

【联想】acceleration n. 加速，加快

【例句】Growth will accelerate to 2.9 per cent next year.

【译文】明年的增长会加速至 2.9%。

acceptance [ək'septəns]　n. 接受，接纳；承认

【联想】accept vt. 接受；acceptable a. 可接受的

access ['ækses]　n. 通路，访问 vt. 访问；存取

【搭配】get/gain/have (no) access to (没) 有机会或权利得到 (接近、进入、使用)

【联想】accessible a. 可接近的

【例句】Yet these latter individuals generally lack access to any specialty care.

【译文】但是后者通常情况下没有获得专业护理的机会。

accidental [ˌæksi'dentl]　a. 意外的，偶然 (发生) 的

【联想】accident n. 事故

【例句】This ensures that concurrent updates to an item do not result in accidental data loss.

【译文】这确保了对项目的并发更新不会导致意外的数据丢失。

accomplish [əˈkʌmplɪʃ]　　　　　v. 完成，实现，达到

【联想】accomplishment n. 成就，成绩

【例句】I accomplished two hours' work before dinner.

【译文】我在吃晚饭前完成了两小时的工作。

accord [əˈkɔːd]　　　　　v. 给予；允许；使一致

【搭配】according to 按照，根据；据……所说，
按……所载

【联想】accordingly ad. 依照；由此，于是；相应地

【例句】His opinion accorded with mine.

【译文】他的意见与我的一致。

account [əˈkaunt] vi. (数量上、比例上) 占；解释
　　　　　　　　　　　n. 账，账户，说明，叙述

【搭配】account for 解释；on account of 因为，由于；
on no account 决不；on all accounts 无论如
何；take into account 考虑，重视

【例句】The energy consumed by buildings already accounts for around 45% of greenhouse-gas e-
missions.

【译文】建筑消耗的能源已经占据了温室气体排放量的
45% 左右。

accumulate [əˈkjuːmjəleit]　　　　v. 积累；积聚；
　　　　　　　　　　(数量) 逐渐增加；(数额) 逐渐增长

【例句】By investing wisely she accumulated a fortune.

【译文】她投资精明，累积了一笔财富。

accurate ['ækjurit]   *a*. 正确的，精确的

【联想】accuracy *n*. 精确，精准

【例句】Although technically accurate, that is an impersonal assessment.

【译文】虽然从技术上说是精确的，但那是一个不讲人情的评估。

ache [eik]   *n*. （身体某部位的）疼痛
                          vi. 疼痛；隐痛

【例句】Muscular aches and pains can be soothed by a relaxing massage.

【译文】放松按摩可以缓解肌肉疼痛。

achievement [ə'tʃiːvmənt]
                    n. 完成，达到；成就，成绩

【联想】achieve *vt*. 达到，取得

【例句】Conquest of rabies would be recognized as a great achievement to the work of science.

【译文】攻克狂犬病会被认为是科学研究的一项伟大成就。

acid ['æsid]   *n*. 酸 *a*. 酸的

【联想】acidify *vt*. 酸化

acknowledge [ək'nɔlidʒ]

vt. 承认；感谢；告知收到（信件等）

【联想】acknowledgement *n.* 承认，感谢

【例句】I acknowledge the truth of his statement.

【译文】我承认他说的是事实。

acquire [ə'kwaiə]

vt. 取得，获得；学到

【联想】acquisition *n.* 获得，得到

【例句】Most adults find it extremely difficult to acquire even a basic knowledge, particularly in a short time.

【译文】多数成人发现，即使学会一种基本知识也是非常困难的，尤其是在很短的时间内。

activity [æk'tiviti]

n. 活动；活力；行动

activate ['æktiveit]

vt. 使活动起来，使开始

【例句】Research discovered that plants infected with a virus give off a gas that activates disease resistance in neighboring plants.

【译文】研究发现，感染了病毒的植物会释放出一种气体，来激活周围植物的疾病抵抗能力。

【导学】近义词：stimulate，initiate，arouse，actuate

adapt [ə'dæpt]

vt. 使适应；改编

【搭配】adapt oneself to 使自己适应或习惯于某事

adapt...to 使……适应

【联想】 adaptive *a*. 适应的；adaptation *n*. 改编，适应

【例句】 They want to facilitate their children to adapt to nursery at the age of about three.

【译文】 他们想帮助孩子在三岁左右适应托儿所的生活。

addict [ə'dikt]　　　　　*vt*. 使成瘾，热衷于
　　　　　　　　　　　　　n. 瘾君子，吸毒成瘾的人

【搭配】 be addicted to 对……上瘾

【联想】 addictive *a*. 成瘾的；addiction *n*. 瘾

【例句】 By this reasoning, early humans then became addicted to fruit, and any gene that helped them to find it was selected for.

【译文】 根据这个推理，早期人类对水果上瘾，任何帮助他们找到水果的基因都是被选择的。

addition [ə'diʃən]　　　　　*n*. 加，加法
　　　　　　　　　　　　　　附加部分，增加（物）

【搭配】 in addition 另外；in addition to 除……之外

【联想】 additional *a*. 附加的，另外的

adequate ['ædikwit]　　　　　*a*. 足够的，充分的

【例句】 You are bound to have nights where you don't get an adequate amount of sleep.

【译文】 你一定会经历睡眠不足的夜晚的。

adjust [ə'dʒʌst]　　　　　*v.* 调整，调节；校准；适应

【搭配】adjust...to 使……适应于

【联想】adjustment *n.* 调整，调节

【例句】He adjusts what he does according to what his daily readings tell him about his condition.

【译文】他根据自己每日阅读的状况来调整自己的行为。

Day 2

administer [əd'ministə] *vt.* 管理，经营；行政机关

【联想】administration *n.* 管理

【例句】In the 3rd International Mathematics and Science Study，13-year-olds from Singapore achieved the best scores in standardized tests of maths and science that were administered to 287,896 students from 41 countries.

【译文】在第三届国际数学与科学研究中，来自新加坡的13岁年龄组在数学和科学标准化考试中获得最好成绩，参加该项测试的共有来自41个国家的287896名学生。

admonish [əd'mɔniʃ]

v. 责备；告诫；警告；力劝；忠告

【例句】They admonished me for taking risks with my health.

【译文】他们责备我不应拿自己的健康冒险。

adopt [ə'dɔpt] *vt.* 采用，采纳；收养；通过

【搭配】the adopted children 收养的孩子

【联想】adoption *n.* 采纳；收养

【例句】 Since pollution control measures tend to be money consuming, many industries hesitate to adopt them.

【译文】 因为污染控制措施会增加开销，所以很多行业在采取这些措施时都很犹豫。

adult [ə'dʌlt, 'ædʌlt]   *n*. 成人 *a*. 成年的；成熟的

【联想】 adulthood *n*. 成年人

【例句】 Given that we can not turn the clock back, adults can still do plenty to help the next generation cope.

【译文】 虽然我们不能让时光倒流，但成年人仍能够做很多事情帮助下一代应对。

advance [əd'vɑːns]   *n*./*v*. 前进，行进；进步；进展；（价格、价值的）上涨，提高

【联想】 advanced *a*. 先进的，高级的

advantage [əd'vɑːntidʒ]   *n*. 优点，有利条件；利益，好处

【搭配】 take advantage of 乘……之机，利用
　　　　be of advantage to 利于

advertise ['ædvətaiz]   *vt*. 做广告

【联想】 advertisement *n*. 广告

【搭配】 advertise for 为……广而告之

11

【例句】If I were to advertise for sleepwalkers for an experiment，I doubt that I'd get many takers.

【译文】如果我要招募梦游者做试验，我觉得可能不会有很多人接受。

advocate ['ædvəkət]　　　　*n*. 提倡者，鼓吹者
　　　　　['ædvəkeit]　　　　*vt*. 提倡，鼓吹

【例句】Its advocates point out that the ability to identify untrustworthy people should be favored evolutionally.

【译文】其拥护者们认为，从进化的角度来看，识别不值得信任的人的能力应该受到青睐。

aerobic [eə'rəubik]　　*a*. 需氧的；好氧的；有氧的；增强心肺功能的

【例句】Aerobic exercise can do good to people both mentally and physically.

【译文】有氧运动对人的身心都有益处。

aesthetic [iːs'θetik]　　*a*. 美学的，审美的；悦目的，雅致的

【例句】The more one is conscious of one's political bias，the more chance one has of acting politically without sacrificing one's aesthetic and intellectual integrity.

【译文】越是意识到自己的政治态度，就越可能按政治行事而同时又不牺牲自己美学和思想上的气节。

affect [ə'fekt] *vt.* 影响，作用；使感动；(疾病) 侵袭

【例句】In conclusion，using a computer，particularly for extended periods，may affect the parent-children in families.

【译文】总之，使用电脑，尤其是长时间使用电脑，可能会影响家庭亲子关系。

affection [ə'fekʃən] *n.* 爱，感情；作用，影响

【搭配】have an affection for sb. 热爱某人

【例句】We know the kiss as a form of expressing affection.

【译文】我们知道亲吻是表达感情的一种方式。

afford [ə'fɔːd] *v.* 承担得起 (后果)；负担得起；提供；买得起；(有时间) 做，能做；给予

【联想】affordable *a.* 负担得起的，可承受的

【例句】We cannot afford to ignore this warning.

【译文】我们对这个警告绝不能等闲视之。

agency ['eidʒənsi] *n.* 代理 (处)，代办 (处)

【例句】The agency developed a campaign that fo-

cused on travel experiences such as freedom，
escape，relaxation and enjoyment of the
great western outdoors.

【译文】 这个代理商开展了一项活动，重点关注旅行体
验，如在广阔的西部户外旅行的自由、逃离现
实的生活、放松和乐趣。

---

agenda [əˈdʒendə]　　　　　　　*n*. 议事日程，记事册

【搭配】 put on the agenda 提到议事日程上来

---

agent [ˈeidʒənt]　　　　　　　*n*. 代理人；经办人

【例句】 The agent stressed the need to fulfill the
order exactly.

【译文】 代理人强调要严格按照要求完成订单。

---

aggravate [ˈægrəveit]　　　　　　*vt*. 加重；加剧；
　　　　　　　　　　　　　　　使恼火，激怒；使……恶化

---

aggression [əˈɡreʃən]　　　　　　*n*. 侵略，攻击

【联想】 aggressive *a*. 侵略的，侵犯的

---

aid [eid]　　　　　　　　　　*vi*. 援助，救援
　　　　　　　　　　　　　n. 援助，救护；助手，辅助物

【导学】 辨析 aid，assist，help：做动词时，aid 指提供

帮助、支援或救助；assist 指"给……帮助"或"支持"，尤指作为隶属或补充；help 的含义较多，表示"给予协助、救助，对……有帮助，（在商店或餐馆中）为……服务，促进，（治疗、药物等）缓解、减轻（疼痛、病症）"；help 为普通词，常可代替 aid、assist。做名词时，aid 指帮助的行为或结果，也指助人者，辅助设备；assist 指助人行为；help 指帮助的行动或实例，或指补救的办法，也指助手、雇工。

【例句】Researchers at University of Chicago Pritzker School of Medicine presented data on a CAD (computer-aided diagnosis) program.

【译文】芝加哥大学普利兹克医学院的研究人员展示了 CAD（计算机辅助诊断）程序的数据。

ailment [ˈeilmənt]　　　　　　　*n.* 小病；轻病；小恙

【联想】ail *vi.* 生病

【例句】A surprising number of ailments are caused by unsuspected environmental factors.

【译文】有大量疾病是由不明环境因素造成的。

alarm [əˈlɑːm]　　　　　　*vt.* 惊动，惊吓；向……报警
　　　　　　　　　　　　　　　n. 惊恐；警报；警报器

【例句】The pace of urbanization is being accelerated

at an alarming rate.

【译文】城镇化的步伐正在以惊人的速度加快。

alcohol [ˈælkəhɒl]   *n*. 酒精，乙醇

【联想】alcoholic *a*. 含有乙醇的，含有酒精的 *n*. 酒鬼，酗酒者

【例句】Alcohol in excess is still bad for you，but a glass of wine with dinner is probably fine for nonalcoholics.

【译文】过量饮酒对你仍然有害，不过晚餐时喝一杯酒对非嗜酒者恐怕无害。

alert [əˈlɜːt]   *n*. 警惕 *a*. 警觉的
                                              vt. 使警觉；使意识到

【例句】The scientist is then constantly on the alert for new paths to take in his or her work.

【译文】然后，科学家一直对其工作中采取的新路径保持警惕。

alien [ˈeiljən]   *a*. 外国的，外国人的；陌生的；
                                  性质不同的，不相容的

【导学】alien 与 foreigner 都含有"外国人"的意思。alien 指住在一个国家，但不是该国公民的人；foreigner 指生于或来自他国者，尤指有

不同语言、文化的人。

【例句】We deport aliens who slip across our borders.

【译文】我们把偷渡入境的外国人驱逐出境。

allergy ['æləʤi]　　　　　　　*n*. 过敏；变态反应

【联想】allergic *a*. 过敏的

alleviate [ə'liːvieit]

vt. 减轻（痛苦等），缓和（情绪）

【例句】The doctor gave him an injection in order to alleviate the pain.

【译文】医生给他注射来减轻疼痛。

allocate ['æləkeit]　　　　　*vt*. 分配；拨……（给）；
　　　　　　　　　　　　　　　　划……（归）

【例句】More resources are being allocated to the project.

【译文】正在调拨更多的资源给这个项目。

alternate ['ɔːltəneit]　　　　　*v*. 交替，轮流
　　　　　['ɔːltə:neit]　　　　　　*n*. 代替者；代理人

【导学】近义词：vary, fluctuate, vacillate, oscillate, waver, seesaw, teeter, shift, sway, totter; rotate, substitute

【例句】Conversation calls for a willingness to alternate the role of speaker with that of listener, and it calls for occasional "digestive pauses" by both.

【译文】会话要求说话人与听话人都愿意交换角色，并且需要双方偶尔做出"消化停顿"以理解彼此的意思。

alternative [ɔːl'təːnətiv]　　　　　*a.* 两者选一的
　　　　　　　　　　　　　　　　　n. 供选择的东西；取舍

【例句】Now it is time to start thinking about the long-term effects of alternative energy sources.

【译文】现在是时候开始考虑可代替能源的长期效应了。

alter ['ɔːltə]　　　　　　　　　　*vt.* 改变，变更

【导学】辨析 alter，change，convert，modify，shift，transform，vary：alter 指局部、表面的改变，不影响事物的本质或总体结构，如修改衣服的大小等；change 指全部、完全的改变；convert 指由一种形式或用途变为另一种形式或用途；modify 指变小的修改，只能用于改变方法、计划、制度、组织、意思、条款等；shift 指位置或方向的移动、改变；transform 指外貌、性格或性质的彻底改变；vary 多指形式、外表、本质上的繁多而断续的变化或

改变，使其多样化。

【例句】 With the tools of technology man has altered many physical features of the Earth.

【译文】 通过一些技术手段，人类已经改变了地球的许多物理特征。

amaze [əˈmeiz]　　　　　　　　*vt.* 使惊愕，使惊叹

【导学】 辨析 amaze，astonish，surprise，shock：前三个词中，amaze 语气最强，尤其在被认为不可能之事实际上已发生时使用，也可表示"惊奇，惊叹"；astonish 语气稍强，意为"使大吃一惊，使惊愕"，指事情的发生不可思议而"难以置信"；surprise 是一般用语，指对事出突然或出乎意料而"吃惊，惊奇"；shock 意为"使……震惊，使……惊讶"，指事物的发生出乎意料，使人感到震惊。

amazing [əˈmeiziŋ]　　*a.* 令人惊讶的，令人吃惊的

【导学】 It's amazing that... 从句中的动词用原形或"should＋原形"表示虚拟语气。

【例句】 Some people apparently have an amazing ability to come up with the right answer.

【译文】 很明显，一些人有惊人的得出正确答案的能力。

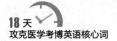
Day 3

ambition [æmˈbiʃən]　　　　　　　　*n*. 雄心；野心

【联想】ambitious *a*. 野心勃勃的

【例句】Not just on the opportunities that will open up to them and only be limited by their own ambition and abilities.

【译文】不是取决于他们将面临的机会，而是只限于他们自己的野心和能力。

amount [əˈmaunt]　　　　　　*n*. 数据，数额，总数
　　　　　　　　　　　　　vt.（to）合计，相当于，等同

【搭配】a large amount of（＋不可数名词）大量的

【导学】辨析 number, total, amount：number 和 total 均为及物动词；amount 是不及物动词，须加 to 再跟宾语。

【例句】Getting a proper amount of rest is absolutely essential for increasing your energy.

【译文】适量的休息绝对是增加体能所必需的。

amplify [ˈæmplifai]　　　　　　*vt*. 放大，增大，扩大

【例句】By turning this knob to the right you can

amplify the sound from the radio.

【译文】 朝右边拧一拧这个旋钮，你就能放大收音机的
声音。

analysis [əˈnælisis]   *n.* 分析，解析

【联想】 analyst *n.* 分析者；analytical *a.* 分析的；
analyse/-ze *vt.* 分析

【导学】 该词复数形式为 analyses。
单复数形式转换：
basis—bases 基础
crisis—crises 危机
thesis—theses 论题
hypothesis—hypotheses 假设
diagnosis—diagnoses 诊断
emphasis—emphases 强调

anatomy [əˈnætəmi] *n.* 解剖学；(动植物的)结构；解剖

【例句】 The beauty of the device is that it contributes
to the evolution of human anatomy.

【译文】 这个设备的优点就在于它有助于人类解剖学的
发展。

ancient [ˈeinʃənt]   *a.* 古代的，古老的

【例句】 Floods have undermined the foundation of the
ancient bridge.

【译文】 洪水已经侵蚀了古老桥梁的根基。

anesthetic [ˌænəsˈθetik]　　　　　　*a*. 麻醉的

annoy [əˈnɔi]　　　　　*vt*. 使烦恼，使生气，打搅

【例句】 Although she is frequently annoyed when I try to gather what I consider basic information，I know she is also relieved that someone is watching out for her.

【译文】 尽管当我搜集我认为的基础信息时她常感觉恼火，但我知道她也会感觉安心，因为有人在照看着她。

annual [ˈænjuəl] *a*. 每年的，年度的 *n*. 年刊，年鉴

【联想】 daily *n*. 日刊；weekly *n*. 周刊；monthly *n*. 月刊；quarterly *n*. 季刊；yearly/annual *n*. 年刊

【例句】 The fruit accounted for more than half the country's annual exports，according to a recent report.

【译文】 根据最新的报告，这种水果的出口量占该国年度出口总量的一半以上。

anti- [ˌænti]　　　　　　　　　　　*prefix* 反，逆

【联想】 antibody 抗体；antibiotic 抗生素；antidepressant 抗抑郁药物；antioxidant 抗氧化剂；antiretroviral 抗逆转录病毒的

anticipate [æn'tisipeit]　　　　　 *v*. 预料，预计

【例句】It is anticipated that inflation will stabilize at 3%.

【译文】据预测，通货膨胀将稳定在3%。

anxiety [æŋ'zaiəti]　　　　 *n*. 挂念，焦虑，担心；
　　　　　　　　　　　　　　　　　　渴望，热望

【联想】anxious *a*. 焦虑的

【例句】He was waiting for his brother's return with anxiety.

【译文】他焦急地等着兄弟归来。

apart [ə'pɑːt]　　　　 *ad*. 分离，隔开；相距，相隔

【搭配】apart from（= besides）除……之外

【联想】except for 除……之外；in addition to 除……之外；fall apart 土崩瓦解

apology [ə'pɒlədʒi]　　　　　 *n*. 道歉，歉意

【搭配】make an apology to sb. for (doing) sth. 为某事向某人道歉

【联想】apologize *v*. 道歉

appalling [ə'pɔːliŋ]　　　 *a*. 骇人听闻的，令人震惊的，
　　　　　　　　　　　　　　　　　　可怕的

apparent [ə'pærənt]　　　　　　*a.* 明显的；表面的

【搭配】 apparent to 对……是显而易见的

【例句】 It is apparent that the watches that finally arrived have been produced from inferior materials.

【译文】 很明显，最后到货的那批手表是用劣等材料制成的。

appeal [ə'piːl]　　　　　*vi.* (to) 请求，呼吁；吸引；

　　　　　　　　　　　　n. 呼吁；吸引力；上诉；求助

【例句】 On the positive side, emotional appeals may respond to a consumer's real concerns.

【译文】 从积极的方面来说，（广告的）情感鼓动可能反映消费者真正的需求。

appetite ['æpitait]　　　　　*n.* 食欲，胃口；欲望

【搭配】 have no appetite for work 不想工作

【联想】 have a desire for, have inclination for, long for, be hungry/thirsty for 渴望

appliance [ə'plaiəns]　　　*n.* 用具，设备，器械；装置

【联想】 equipment *n.* 设备（不可数）；instrument *n.* 仪器；facilities *n.* 设施

apply [ə'plai]　　　　　　*vi.* 申请 *vt.* 运用，应用

【搭配】 apply for 申请；apply... to 将……应用于，

涂，抹；apply oneself to（doing）sth. 致力于
【联想】application *n*. 申请；applicant *n*. 申请人
【例句】I want to apply for the job.
【译文】我想申请这项工作。

appoint [əˈpɔint]　　　　　　　*vt*. 任命，委派；约定

【搭配】appoint sb.（后面接名词）任命某人
【联想】appointment *n*. 任命，委派
【例句】Make an appointment to see Mr. Okes，and I'll write to him and to your doctor.
【译文】和奥克斯先生预约吧，并且我会给他和你的医生写信。

appreciate [əˈpriːʃieit]　　　*vt*. 感激，感谢；评价；
　　　　　　　　　　　　　　　　　　欣赏，赏识

【导学】后面接动名词，不接动词不定式，如：appreciate（one's）doing.
【例句】I appreciate President Castro's invitation for us to visit Cuba，and have been delighted with the hospitality we have received since arriving here.
【译文】我感谢卡斯特罗主席邀请我们访问古巴。我们来到这里后受到了热情接待，使我一直沉浸在喜悦之中。

approach [əˈprəutʃ]　　　　　*n*. 靠近；方法；要求
　　　　　　　　　　　　　　　　　v. 接近 *vt*. 处理；对待

【搭配】approach to = access to 接近

【例句】They must change their institutional and legal approaches to water use.

【译文】他们必须从制度和法规的方式上改变对水资源的使用。

appropriate [əˈprəupriət]   *a.* 适当的，恰当的

【搭配】be appropriate to 对……适合

【导学】It's appropriate that... 从句中的谓语动词用原形或 "should + 原形"。

【例句】It will be an indication that you are starting to get an appropriate amount of sleep at night.

【译文】这将表明你正在进入夜间睡眠适量的时期。

approve [əˈpruːv]   *v.* 赞成，赞许，同意；批准，审议，通过

【搭配】approve sth. 批准某事

approve of sth. 赞许、同意某事

approve of sb. doing sth. 同意某人做某事

【联想】approval *n.* 赞成，赞许

【例句】Mike Foster is trying to get Parliament to approve a new law.

【译文】迈克·福斯特正努力使国会通过一项新的法律。

Day 4

approximate [ə'prɔksimeit]　　　*a*. 大致的，近似的

【联想】approximately *ad*. 大约，粗略地（近义词：roughly）

【例句】Approximately how many Americans suffer chronic insomnia?

【译文】大约有多少美国人患有慢性失眠症?

archaeology [ˌɑːkiˈɔlədʒi]　　　*n*. 考古学

architect ['ɑːkitekt]　　*n*. 建筑师；设计师；缔造者

【联想】architecture *n*. 建筑；建筑学

argument ['ɑːgjumənt]　　*n*. 争论，辩论；论点，依据

【联想】argue *v*. 争论

【例句】There are two bad arguments for banning such labels.

【译文】关于禁止此类标签有两个错误的理由。

arrogant ['ærəgənt]　　　　*a*. 傲慢的，自大的

【联想】arrogancy *n*. 傲慢

【例句】Often these children realize that they know

more than their teachers, and their teachers
often feel that these children are arrogant,
inattentive, or unmotivated.

【译文】这些孩子常常觉得他们比老师知道的要多，老师们常常感到这些孩子自大、不用心或者缺乏学习动机。

artificial [ˌɑːtiˈfiʃəl]　　　　　a. 人工的，人造的；人为的，做作的

【导学】辨析 artificial，fake，false：artificial 指由人工制成的而非自然的；fake 指"伪造的，冒充的"；false 是指与真理或事实相反的，故意造假的。

【例句】The colors in these artificial flowers are guaranteed not to come out.

【译文】这些假花保证不会褪色。

aspect ['æspekt]　　　　　n. 方面；样子，面貌

【联想】respect v. 尊敬；inspect v. 视察；prospect n. 前景；expect v. 期望；perspective n. 洞察力

【例句】Most national news has an important financial aspect to it.

【译文】绝大多数的国内新闻都会涉及重要的金融信息。

aspirin ['æspərin]　　　　　n. 阿司匹林

aspiration [ˌæspəˈreiʃən] *n*. 强烈的愿望，志向，抱负

【例句】 But as useful as computers are, they are no-where close to achieving anything remotely resembling these early aspirations for human-like behavior.

【译文】 但是，尽管计算机非常有用，但它们离实现早期期望的类似人类行为的愿望还差之万里。

assassination [əˌsæsiˈneiʃən] *n*. 暗杀，刺杀

【联想】 assassinate *vt*. 暗杀，行刺

【例句】 Two members of a UN team investigating the February assassination of former Lebanese Prime Minister on Friday interviewed Lebanon's President.

【译文】 周五，负责调查黎巴嫩前总理二月遭暗杀事件的两名联合国调查小组成员采访了黎巴嫩总统。

assert [əˈsəːt] *vt*. 宣称，断言；维护，坚持（权利等）

【例句】 Why does the author assert that all things from American are fascinating to foreigners? Because they have gained much publicity through American media?

【译文】 为什么作者断言美国所有的东西对国外人都有吸引力？因为它们通过美国的媒体已经获得了巨大的知名度吗？

assimilate [əˈsimileit]　　　*vt.* 吸收，消化；使同化

　　　　　　　　　　　　　　　　　　vi. 同化，融入

【例句】One of the reasons why children resemble their parents is that they assimilate the characteristics of their parents.

【译文】孩子长得像父母，其原因之一就是孩子吸取并同化了父母的各种特征。

assess [əˈses]　*vt.* 估计，估算；评估，评价，评定

【联想】access *n.* 接近；excess *n.* 超额量；asset *n.* 资产

【导学】辨析 assess，estimate，evaluate：assess 为征税估定（财产）的价值，确定或决定（某项付费，如税或罚款）的金额，评估某事物的价值、意义或程度；estimate 估计，恰当地推测；evaluate 确定……的数值或价值，对……评价，仔细地考察和判断。

【例句】Treatment outcome was initially assessed at one year, with up to 10 years of follow-up evaluations.

【译文】治疗结果最初是一年评估一次，并有长达十年的随访评估。

assist [əˈsist]　　　　　　　　　　　*vi.* 援助，帮助

【联想】assistance *n.* 帮助，援助

【搭配】assist in doing sth. 帮助做某事

assist sb. in doing sth. 帮助某人做某事

assist sb. to do sth. 帮助某人做某事

【例句】The clerk assisted the judge by looking up related precedent.

【译文】这位书记官协助那位法官查阅相关的判决先例。

associate [əˈsəuʃieit]　　　*vt.* 联系；联合 *vi.* 交往

n. 合作人，同事

【搭配】associate... with 把……与……联系在一起

【联想】association *n.* 协会，团体；交往；联合，合伙；

associate... with, link... to, relate... with/to,

combine/connect... with 把……与……联系在

一起；have association with 与……交往

【例句】What do you associate with such heavy snow?

【译文】这样一场大雪，你联想到什么？

assume [əˈsjuːm]　　　*vt.* 假定，设想；假装；承担

【联想】consume *v.* 消费；presume *v.* 推测；resume

v. 重新开始；assumption *n.* 假定，设想；

担任，承当；假装

【例句】Researchers conclude that any effect of money on happiness is smaller than most daydreamers assume.

【译文】研究者得出结论，金钱对幸福的影响程度要比大多数空想家假设的程度小。

assure [əˈʃuə]　　　　　　　　*vt.* 使确信；向……保证

【导学】辨析 assure，ensure：两者皆意为"保证"，但用法有些区别，具体用法有 assure sb. that/assure sb. of；ensure that/ensure sb. against/from；assure/ensure sth.。

【联想】insure *v.* 保险，投保；assurance *n.* 保证

【例句】By the new study the technique helps the scientists assure the depth of anesthesia during surgery.

【译文】通过这项新的研究，该技术有助于科学家确保手术期间麻醉的深度。

athlete [ˈæθliːt]　　　　　　　*n.* 运动员，运动选手

【联想】athletic *a.* 运动的，体育的，运动员的

atmosphere [ˈætməsfiə]　　*n.* 空气；大气，大气层；气氛

ultimate [ˈʌltimit]　　*a.* 最后的，最终的 *n.* 终极，顶点

【例句】The union leaders declared that the ultimate aim of their struggle was to increase pay and improve working conditions for the workers.

【译文】工会领导人宣称，他们斗争的最终目的是要增加工人工资和改善工人的工作条件。

undergo [ˌʌndəˈgəu]　　　　　　*vt.* 经历，遭受

【搭配】undergo hardships/changes 经历苦难/变化

【导学】在英文中有许多以 under- 这个前缀开头的单词，多指"在……之下"。

【例句】Security programs should undergo actuarial review.

【译文】保障方案应经过精算评估。

undergraduate [ˌʌndəˈgrædjuit]

n. 大学生，大学肄业生

【联想】undergraduate *n.* 本科生；postgraduate *n.* 研究生；PhD student 博士生

understanding [ˌʌndəˈstændiŋ] *n.* 理解，理解力；谅解
a. 能体谅人的，宽容的

【例句】Developers hope the project will increase Germans' understanding of China and Chinese culture.

【译文】开发者们希望这个项目能增加德国人对中国及其文化的理解。

undertake [ˌʌndəˈteik]　　　*vt.* 承担，接收；
约定，保证；着手，从事

【联想】undertaking *n.* 任务，项目；事业，企业；承诺，保证；殡仪业

【搭配】undertake to do/that 答应做

undertake an attack 发动进攻

undertake a great effort 做出巨大努力

【例句】This newly established fund has a range of medical programs undertaken by universities, industrial labs, or university-industry collaborative projects.

【译文】这个新成立的基金有一系列由大学、工业实验室或大学－工业合作项目承担的医疗项目。

uneasy [ʌn'iːzi]   a. 不安的，忧虑的

【联想】uneasiness n. 不安，焦虑

近义词为 nervous。

【例句】He was particularly uneasy about being unable to isolate the rabic substance.

【译文】他对无法分离出狂犬病物质感到特别不安。

unfortunately [ʌn'fɔːtʃənətli]   ad. 恐怕，不幸的是

unique [juː'niːk]   a. 唯一的，独一无二的

【搭配】be unique to... 对……来说是独一无二的

【例句】Each United States Surgeon General has the unique opportunity to create his or her own lasting legacy.

【译文】每位美国卫生部长都有独特的机会让自己流芳百世。

universal [ˌjuːnɪˈvəːsəl]　　　*a*. 普遍的；宇宙的，全世界的；普通的，一般的；通用的，万能的

【例句】Personal computers are of universal interest. Everyone is learning how to use them.

【译文】大家都对个人电脑感兴趣，每个人都在学习怎样使用它们。

upper [ˈʌpə]　　　*a*. 上面的，上部的；较高的

【例句】A full moon was beginning to rise and peered redly through the upper edges of fog.

【译文】一轮满月开始升起，带着红色的光芒在雾气上沿朦胧出现。

urban [ˈəːbən]　　　*a*. 城市的，市内的

【例句】Reducing it will require integrated policies for urban planning, transport and housing.

【译文】减少它需要城市规划、交通和住房方面的综合政策。

urge [əːdʒ]　　　*v*./*n*. 强烈希望，竭力主张；鼓励，促进

【搭配】urge sth. on 竭力推荐或力陈某事

【导学】在 urge that... 从句中，谓语动词用原形表示虚拟。

【例句】The urge to survive drove them on.

【译文】求生的欲望促使他们继续努力。

urgent [ˈəːdʒənt]　　　　　　　*a*. 紧迫的；催促的

【例句】It is urgent to modify our relationship with the environment.

【译文】改变我们和环境之间的关系迫在眉睫。

utility [ˈjuːtiliti]　　　　　　*n*. 效用，实用；公用事业

【例句】The abstract shall state briefly the main technical points of the invention or utility model.

【译文】摘要应当简要说明发明或者实用新型的技术要点。

utilize [juːˈtilaiz]　　　　　　　*vt*. 利用，使用

【例句】And they affect how we absorb, utilize and store various nutrients.

【译文】它们影响我们吸收、利用和储存各种营养物质的方式。

utter [ˈʌtə]　　　　　*a*. 完全的，彻底的，绝对的

　　　　　vt. 说，发出（声音）；说出，说明，表达

【搭配】utter one's thoughts/feelings 说出自己的想法/感觉

【例句】What he is doing is utter stupidity!

【译文】他正在做的是完全愚蠢的事！

Day 5

atom [ˈætəm]
n. 原子

【联想】 atomic *a*. 原子的，原子能的

molecule *n*. 分子；particle *n*. 粒子

electron *n*. 电子；nucleus *n*. 原子核

attack [əˈtæk] *n*. 袭击；攻击；抨击，非难；抑制；发作，侵袭；（情感的）一阵突发；（病、虫等的）损害 *v*. 袭击；攻击；（在战争等中使用武器）进攻；抨击；非难；侵袭

【例句】 The school has come under attack for failing to encourage bright pupils.

【译文】 这所学校因未能鼓励聪明学生而受到非难。

attach [əˈtætʃ]
vt. 贴上，系上，附上；使依附

【搭配】 be attached to 喜爱，依恋，附属于

attach importance to 重视……

【联想】 attachment *n*. 附件，依附

【例句】 I've attached my contact information in the recommendation letter.

【译文】 我在推荐信中附上了我的联系方式。

attendance [əˈtendəns]　　　*n*. 出席；出席的人数；
　　　　　　　　　　　　　　　　伺候，照料

attendant [əˈtendənt] *n*. 侍者，服务员；出席者；随从
　　　　　　　　　　a. 出席的；随行的，伴随的

【导学】该词作为形容词不太被大家熟悉，但是形容
　　　　词的词意和用法也要掌握，如：attendant
　　　　problems 随之而来的问题。该词从动词
　　　　attend 派生出来，由于 attend 本身有多层意
　　　　思，所以要将该词与 attend 派生出来的其他
　　　　名词区分开来。

【例句】The Prime Minister was followed by five or
　　　　six attendants when he got off the plane.

【译文】首相从飞机上下来时有五六个随从跟着。

attitude [ˈætitjuːd]　　　　　　　*n*. 态度，看法

attribute [ˈætribjuːt]　　　*vt*. (to) 把……归因于
　　　　　　　　[əˈtribjuːt]　　　*n*. 属性，特征

【搭配】attribute... to... 把……归因于……

【联想】contribute *v*. 贡献；distribute *v*. 分发

【例句】He attributes the U. S. health problems to
　　　　lifestyle factors.

【译文】他将美国人的健康问题归因于生活方式。

author [ˈɔːθə]   *n.* 作者

【导学】 辨析 author，writer：author 指某作品的作者；writer 多指职业性作家。

authority [ɔːˈθɔriti]   *n.* 权力，权威；权威人士；
                                                    (*pl.*) 当局

【例句】 This can lead to a reduction in parental authority.

【译文】 这会导致父母权威受损。

automatic [ˌɔːtəˈmætik]   *a.* 自动的

【例句】 The factory is equipped with two fully automatic assembling lines，and the control room is at the center.

【译文】 这家工厂配备两条全自动生产线，控制室就在正中央。

available [əˈveiləbl]   *a.* 可利用的；可得到的

【导学】 常做表语，做定语要放在所修饰词后面，如：These data are readily available. 这些资料很容易得到。

【例句】 Humanity uses a little less than half the water available worldwide.

【译文】 人类使用了全球可利用水资源的一小部分，不足一半。

average ['ævəridʒ] *a*. 平均的；典型的；正常的；普通的；平常的；一般的 *n*. 平均数；平均水平；一般水准 *v*. 平均为；计算出……的平均数

【例句】40 hours is a fairly average working week for most people.

【译文】对大多数人来说，每周工作 40 小时很正常。

avoid [ə'vɔid] *vt*. 避免，逃避

【搭配】后面接动名词，avoid doing sth. 避免做某事。

【例句】They often try to avoid feeling unpleasant emotions, such as loneliness, worry, and grief.

【译文】他们经常尽量避免产生不愉快的情绪，例如孤独、担心和悲伤。

aware [ə'wɛə] *a*. 知道的，意识到的

【搭配】be aware of 意识到

【例句】Coaches and parents should be aware, at all times, that their feedback to youngsters can greatly affect their children.

【译文】教练和父母要随时意识到他们的反应将会极大地影响到他们的孩子。

awful ['ɔːful] *a*. 糟糕的，极坏的，可怕的

【例句】She had put a good three miles between herself and the awful hitchhiker.

【译文】 她和那个吓人的旅行者之间保持了恰好三英里
的距离。

backlash ['bæklæʃ]　　　　*n.*（对社会变动等的）
　　　　　　　　　　　　　　强烈抵制，集体反对

【例句】 The government is facing an angry backlash
from voters over the new tax.

【译文】 政府正面临选民对新税项的强烈反对。

bacteria [bæk'tiəriə]　　　　　　*n.*（*pl.*）细菌

【联想】 bacterium *n.* 细菌（单数）

【例句】 The bacteria which make the food go bad
prefer to live in the watery regions of the
mixture.

【译文】 能使食物变坏的细菌更喜欢在有水的混合物区
域生存。

balance ['bæləns]　　　　　　　　*vt.* 使平衡
　　　　　　n. 平衡；差额，结余；天平，秤

【搭配】 off balance 不平衡

【例句】 They throw out all ideas about a balanced diet
for the grandkids.

【译文】 他们将孙子、孙女们的均衡饮食思想完全抛于
脑后。

ban [bæn]　　　　　　　　　*n. / vt.* 禁止，取缔

【例句】If the law is passed, wild animals like foxes will be protected under the ban in Britain.

【译文】如果这项法律通过了，像狐狸这样的野生动物在英国就将得到禁令的保护。

bare [beə] *a.* 极少的，仅有的；赤裸的，光秃的，空的

【导学】辨析 bare，blank，empty，hollow，vacant：bare 表示赤裸的，没有通常或适当的覆盖物的；blank 指空白的，未填写的，没有字迹、图像或标记的；empty 指的是无人居住的，内无一物的，未载东西的，还指含义上空洞的；hollow 指中空的，凹的，挖空的；vacant 指空缺的，没有现任者或占有者的。

【例句】We'd better take the bare necessities.

【译文】我们最好只带极少的必需品。

barely ['beəli] *ad.* 仅仅；几乎不能

【联想】seldom/hardly/rarely 几乎不

barrier ['bæriə] *n.* 栅栏；障碍，屏障

【例句】Some people prefer the original English text whereas others feel a translation into their native language removes a barrier to understanding.

【译文】有人更喜欢英语原版文章，也有人觉得翻译成母语消除了理解上的障碍。

basically ['beisikəli]   *ad.* 基本，根本地

basis ['beisis]   *n.* 基础，基底；基准；根据；主要成分（或要素）；（认识论中的）基本原则或原理

【搭配】on the basis of 根据，以……为基础

【导学】该词复数形式为 bases

behave [bi'heiv]   *vi.* 举动，举止，表现

【联想】behaviour *n.* 行为，举止

【搭配】behave oneself 规规矩矩地

【例句】They still seemed to make people behave more honestly.

【译文】他们仍然好像能使人们举止坦诚。

benefit ['benifit]
vt. 对（某人）有用，使受益 *vi.* 得益于
n. 利益，恩惠

【联想】beneficial *a.* 有利的，有益的

【搭配】benefit from 受益于

【例句】Science is supposed to benefit humanity, but because of the conditions under which their tools are made, many scientists may actually be causing harm.

【译文】科学本应造福人类，但由于其工具的制造条件，许多科学家实际上可能会对人类造成伤害。

beverage ['bevəridʒ]　　　　　　　　*n.* 酒水，饮料

【例句】Caffeine in beverages greatly improves performance.

【译文】饮料中的咖啡因会大大提升效能。

biology [bai'ɔlədʒi]　　　　　　　　*n.* 生物学

【例句】The girl shows a special interest in biology.

【译文】这个女孩对生物学表现出特殊的兴趣。

biomarker [ˌbaiəu'ma:kə]　　　　*n.* 生物标志化合物

【例句】Genetic medicine uses genetic or genomic biomarkers in this way.

【译文】遗传医学以这种方式使用遗传或基因组生物标志物。

biomedical [ˌbaiəu'medikəl]　　　*a.* 生物医疗的

【例句】Criticism to the use of animals in biomedical research rests on varied scientific and ethical arguments.

【译文】对在生物医学研究中使用动物的批评是基于各种科学和伦理的角度。

bispectral [bai'spektrəl]　　　　　*a.* 双谱的

【例句】At the same time, bispectral analysis recorded the depth of anesthesia.

【译文】与此同时，双谱分析技术记录了麻醉的深度。

bound [baund]　　　　　　　*a*. 必定，约定；受约束；开往

【搭配】be/feel bound to do sth. 一定；必须；be bound for 准备起程开往……；在赴……途中

【例句】As social workers，general practitioners are bound to constantly contact people in the community.

【译文】作为社会工作者，全科医生必然会经常接触社区中的人。

boundary ['baundəri]　　　　　　　*n*. 界限；边界

【例句】The government will eradicate the boundary for doctors to practice online soon.

【译文】政府很快就会解除医生线上执业的限制。

breakthrough ['breikθru:]　　　　*n*. 重大发现，突破

【导学】来自于词组 break through "突破"。常和 breakdown，outbreak 放在一起考辨析题。outbreak 意思是"（战争的）爆发，（疾病的）发作"。

【例句】While a full understanding of what causes the disease may be several years away，a breakthrough leading to a successful treatment could come much sooner.

【译文】尽管要完全理解这种疾病的病因可能还要好几年时间，但距离治疗方法的突破性进展已为时不远。

tackle ['tækl]　　　　　　　　　*vt.* 解决，处理

【例句】 The problem-behavioral therapy tackles thinking and feeling in a very particular way that medicines may not.

【译文】 问题行为疗法以一种药物无法解决的非常特殊的方式解决了思维和感觉的问题。

tactful ['tæktful]　　　　　*a.* 机智的；老练的，圆滑的

【例句】 The doctor tried to find a tactful way of telling her the truth.

【译文】 医生试图用委婉的方式告诉她真相。

talent ['tælənt]　　　　　　　*n.* 天资；才能；人才

【搭配】 have a talent for 对……有天赋
cultivate/develop one's talent 培养自己的才能

【例句】 They also say that the need for talented, skilled Americans means we have to expand the pool of potential employees.

【译文】 他们也指出对有才华的、技术熟练的美国人的需求，这意味着我们要挖掘员工的潜力。

target ['tɑːgit]　　　　　　　　　*n.* 靶子；目标

【搭配】 hit/miss the target 射中/未射中靶子

【例句】 The Government has set the target for full implementation of whole-day primary schooling for

2007/2008.

【译文】政府已定下目标，将于 2007～2008 学年全面推行全日制小学。

tax [tæks]　　　　　　　　　　　*n.* 税款 *vt.* 征税

【搭配】escape taxes 逃税；collect taxes 征税

【联想】tax-free *a.* 免税的 *ad.* 免税；taxpayer *n.* 纳税人

technician [tekˈnɪʃ(ə)n]　　　*n.* 技术员，技师，技工

technology [tekˈnɒlədʒi]　　*n.* 工业技术，应用科学

【联想】technological *a.* 技术的

【例句】Although science and technology have advanced tremendously over the past century, the Pandemic peril remains.

【译文】尽管科学技术在过去一个世纪里取得了巨大的进步，但大流行的危险依然存在。

teenager [ˈtiːneɪdʒə]　　　*n.* (13～19 岁的) 青少年

【例句】Teenagers who text more than 100 times a day tend to be more shallow.

【译文】每天发短信超过 100 次的青少年往往更为肤浅。

telehealth [ˈtelihelθ]　　　　*n.* 远程医疗

【例句】Henry is just one of a growing number of pioneering patients who are trusting their futures to telehealth.

【译文】亨利只是越来越多的先驱患者中的一员，他们将自己的未来寄托于远程医疗。

telescope ['teliskəup]　　　　　　　　*n*. 望远镜

temper ['tempə]　　　　　　　　*n*. 情绪，脾气

【搭配】be in a good/bad temper 心情好/不好；lose one's temper 发脾气，发怒

【例句】They are ill-tempered.

【译文】他们脾气很糟糕。

temperament ['tempərəmənt]　　　*n*. 气质，性格

【例句】Whether a person likes a routine office job or not depends largely on temperament.

【译文】一个人是否喜欢程式化的办公室工作很大程度上取决于性情。

temporary ['tempərəri]　　　　*a*. 暂时的，临时的

【例句】Their temporary mud huts with thatched roofs of wild grasses often only last six months.

【译文】他们临时搭建的茅草屋顶的小泥屋通常只能维持6个月。

tempt [tempt]　　　　　　*vt*. 引诱，勾引；吸引，
　　　　　　　　　　　　　　引起……的兴趣

【导学】近义词：lure, entice, fascinate, seduce,

appeal to，induce，intrigue，incite，provoke，allure，charm，captivate，stimulate，move，motivate，rouse

【例句】Your offer does not tempt me at all. Nothing can tempt me to leave my present position.

【译文】你的建议一点也打动不了我的心，什么东西都不能诱使我离开现在的职位。

temptation [temp'teiʃən]　　　　*n*. 引诱，诱惑；迷人之物，诱惑物

【例句】It is not easy for us to resist temptation.

【译文】对于我们来说，抵制诱惑是不太容易的。

terminate ['tə:mineit]　　　　*v*. 停止，（使）终止

terminal ['tə:minl]　　　　*a*. 末端的，终点的；期末的；晚期的，致死的
　　　　　　　　　　　　n. 末端；总站；计算机终端

【搭配】terminal cancer 癌症晚期
　　　　terminal heart disease 心脏病晚期

【例句】His mom has a terminal illness.

【译文】他的母亲得了绝症。

therapy ['θerəpi]　　　　*n*. 治疗，疗法

【联想】therapeutic *a*. 治疗的

【例句】Researches show that the most effective treat-

49

ment is the combination of anti-depression and talk therapy.

【译文】研究表明，最有效的治疗方式是抗抑郁和谈话治疗相结合。

threat [θret]   *n.* 威胁，危险现象

threaten ['θretn]   *vt.* 威胁，恐吓

【搭配】threaten sb. with/to do 用……威胁/威胁某人要做

【联想】argue/persuade/talk sb. into doing sth. 说服某人去做某事；cheat/trick sb. into doing sth. 哄骗某人去做某事；force sb. into doing sth. 迫使某人去做某事；frighten/scare/terrify sb. into doing sth. 恐吓某人去做某事；reason sb. into doing sth. 劝说某人去做某事

【例句】It will greatly threaten the security of this country.

【译文】它将会极大地威胁这个国家的安全。

throat [θrəut]   *n.* 喉咙

【搭配】clear one's throat 清喉咙

have a bone in one's throat 难以启齿

tolerate ['tɔləreit]   *vt.* 忍受，容忍，容许

【例句】Women may tolerate small amounts of tobacco worse than men.

【译文】相比男性，女性对少量烟草的耐受度更差。

trace [treis] *n.* 痕迹，踪迹 *vt.* 跟踪，查找

【搭配】trace back to 追溯到

【例句】Much of Chinese mythology is lost，and what is not lost is scattered and difficult to trace.

【译文】中国神话散佚很多，仅存的文献又很分散，难以寻查。

tradition [trə'diʃən] *n.* 传统，惯例

【联想】traditional *a.* 传统的

【例句】Many traditional families are slow to develop personal relationships.

【译文】很多传统家庭在发展人际关系方面比较缓慢。

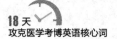
Day 6

calcium [ˈkælsiəm] *n.* 钙

calculate [ˈkælkjuleit] *vt.* 计算，推算；
估计，推测；计划，打算

【联想】calculation *n.* 计算；calculator *n.* 计算器
【例句】The tuition is too high to be calculated.
【译文】学费太高，无法计算了。

calorie [ˈkæləri] *n.* 卡（热量单位）

【例句】I would like to have a cup of black coffee. I am counting my calories at the moment.
【译文】我想要一杯不加糖和奶的咖啡（黑咖啡）。我目前正在控制所摄取的热量。

cancel [ˈkænsəl] *vt.* 取消，撤销；删去

【联想】cancellation *n.* 取消，删除
【例句】All flights having been canceled because of the snowstorm, they decided to take the train.
【译文】因为暴风雪，所有的航班都取消了，他们决定坐火车。

cancer [ˈkænsə] *n.* 癌

【联想】 cancerous *a.* 癌症的

【例句】 Most experts see cancer vaccines as a hybrid of treatment and prevention.

【译文】 大多专家将癌症疫苗看成是治疗和预防的混合体。

candidate ['kændidit]　　*n.* 候选人；报考者；求职者

【例句】 A second language isn't generally required to get a job in business，but having language skills gives a candidate the edge when other qualifications appear to be equal.

【译文】 掌握第二门语言通常不是在贸易方面找到一份工作的条件，但是有语言方面的技能则能使候选人在其他条件同等的情况下比其他人具有更大的优势。

capability [ˌkeipə'biliti] *n.* 能力，才能；性能，容量

【联想】 capable *a.* 能干的，有能力的，有才能的

【搭配】 have the capability of 有 …… 的才能
beyond/above one's capability 超过某人的能力范围

【联想】 have the ability to do，have the capacity for doing/to do 有能力做

capacity [kə'pæsiti]　　　　　*n.* 容量，容积；能力；能量；接受力

【例句】 The memory capacity of bees means they can distinguish among more than 50 different smells to find the one they want.

【译文】 蜜蜂的记忆力意味着它们能在 50 多种不同的味道中找到它们想要的那种。

capture ['kæptʃə]　　　　　 *vt.* 捕获，捉拿；夺得，攻占

【例句】 The decline in moral standards—which has long concerned social analysts—has at last captured the attention of average Americans.

【译文】 被社会学家一直关注的道德滑坡问题，最终引起了美国大众的关注。

carbon ['kɑːbən]　　　　　　　　　　　 *n.* 碳

【例句】 Big challenges still await companies converting carbon dioxide to petrol.

【译文】 巨大的挑战仍然横亘在公司将二氧化碳转化成汽油的道路上。

carbohydrate [ˌkɑːbəu'haidreit]　　　 *n.* 碳水化合物

【例句】 They did eat significantly less fat and slightly fewer carbohydrates.

【译文】 他们确实摄入了明显较少的脂肪和略少一些的碳水化合物。

cardiac ['kɑːdiæk]　　　　　　　　 *a.* 心脏的；心脏病的
　　　　　　　　　　　　　n. 心脏病患者；强心剂；健胃剂

【联想】cardiologist *n*. 心血管医生

【例句】Blocked vessels have several classical symptoms：chest pain，shortness of breath，and abnormal cardiac stress.

【译文】血管堵塞有几个典型的症状：胸痛、呼吸短促和心脏压力异常。

cardiovascular [ˌkɑːdiəʊˈvæskjələ(r)]   *a*. 心血管的

【例句】Women have an advantage to delay over men in terms of cardiovascular disease，like heart attack and stroke.

【译文】在心脏病和中风等心血管疾病方面，女性比男性有延迟患病的优势。

career [kəˈriə]   *n*. 生涯，经历；专业，职业

【例句】A lateral move that hurt my feelings and blocked my professional progress，promoted me to abandon my relatively high profile career.

【译文】一次侧面的打击伤害了我的感情，阻碍了我事业的发展，使我放弃了我那份引人注目的工作。

casual [ˈkæʒjuəl]   *a*. 随便的；偶然的；临时的

【例句】Friendships among Americans tend to be casual.

【译文】美国人之间的友谊往往是比较随意的。

catastrophe [kəˈtæstrəfi]　　　　　*n*. 大灾难，大祸

【联想】catastrophic *a*. 灾难的

【例句】Influenza appears to have all the ingredients for another catastrophic pandemic.

【译文】流感似乎具有另一场灾难性大流行病的所有因素。

【导学】　近义词：disaster，calamity，mishap，mischance，misadventure，failure，fiasco，misery，accident，trouble，casualty，misfortune，infliction，affliction，contretemps，stroke，havoc，ravage，wreck，fatality，grief，crash，devastation，desolation，avalanche，hardship，blow，visitation，ruin，reverse，emergency，scourge，cataclysm，convulsion，debacle，tragedy，adversity，bad luck，upheaval

catalog [ˈkætəlɔg]　　　　*vt*. 将……编入目录 *n*. 目录

【联想】近义词 catalogue

【例句】It is tested, processed, packaged, catalogued, marketed and sold.

【译文】它被测试、加工、包装、编目、营销和售出。

category [ˈkætigəri]　　　　　*n*. 种类，类别；（逻）范畴

【例句】Freud should be placed in the same category as Darwin.

【译文】弗洛伊德应该与达尔文归为同一类。

caution [ˈkɔːʃən]　　　　　　　　　*n.* 谨慎，小心；警告

　　　　　　　　　　　　　　　　　　vt. 警告，提醒

【联想】cautious *a.* 谨慎的，小心的

【搭配】do sth. with caution 谨慎小心地做

　　　　caution sb. against/about sth. 警告某人某事

【例句】Others viewed the findings with caution，noting that a cause-and-effect relationship between passive smoking and cancer remains to be shown.

【译文】其他人谨慎地看待这些发现，因为他们注意到在被动吸烟和癌症之间的因果关系仍然有待观察。

cervical [ˈsɜːvɪkl]　　　　　　　　　　　*a.* 宫颈的

【例句】It's true that the U.S. Food and Drug Administration，has approved vaccines against cervical and liver cancer.

【译文】美国食品和药物管理局（U.S. Food and Drug Administration）确实批准了预防宫颈癌和肝癌的疫苗。

challenge [ˈtʃælɪndʒ]　　　　　　　*vt.* 向……挑战

　　　　　　　　　　　　　　n. 挑战，挑战书；艰巨任务，难题

【搭配】challenge sb. to do sth. 向某人挑战做某事

　　　　challenge sb. to sth. 向某人挑战某事

【例句】Genetic medicine poses great challenges to

medical practice.

【译文】 遗传医学对医疗实践提出了巨大的挑战。

change [tʃeindʒ] *vt*. 改变，变更，变革；交换，更迭，替换；把……变成……（into）*n*. 改变，变化；找回的零钱；调换（口味）；换衣服

【联想】 changeable *a*. 可交换的

【例句】 Doctors' role and responsibilities change all the time.

【译文】 医生的角色和职责一直都在改变。

character ['kæriktə] *n*. 性格，品质；特性，特征；人物，角色；（书写或印刷）符号，（汉）字

【导学】 辨析 character, nature, personality：character 指性格、品性、人格，尤指是非观念、品德等；nature 指性格、天性、气质等的总称，与生俱来的，也指事物的性质或人类的通性；personality 指个性、个人魅力，强调感情因素。

characteristic [ˌkæriktə'ristik] *n*. 特征，特性 *a*. 特有的，独特的

【导学】 辨 析 characteristic, feature, property, quality：characteristic 指人、物的抽象特点或特征，是识别他人或他物的明显标志；feature 指非常突出的特点，具有足以引人

注目的部分或细节，常用于生理、自然条件、物品等；property 性质、特征，通常指事物的基本特征；quality 指个人的品行、品质。

【例句】The molecular characteristics of a disorder or the genetic make-up of an individual can fine tune a diagnosis and inform its management.

【译文】疾病的分子特征或个体的基因构成可以微调诊断并为其管理提供信息。

characterize [ˈkærɪktəraɪz]   *vt.* 描绘……的特性，刻画……的性格

【例句】Our society is characterized with the "knowledge economy".

【译文】我们的社会以"知识经济"为特征。

cheat [tʃiːt]   *vt.* 哄骗，骗取 *vi.* 作弊，欺诈 *n.* 欺骗，骗子

【搭配】cheat sb.（out）of sth. 骗取某人的某物
cheat sb. into the belief that 哄骗某人相信

【导学】辨析 cheat，deceive：cheat 指用诡计欺骗，骗取；deceive 表示误导，使……相信不真实的情况，做出错误的判断。

【例句】People are extraordinarily skilled at spotting cheats.

【译文】人们非常擅长发现骗子。

chemical ['kemikəl]　　　　　　　　*a*. 化学的
　　　　　　　　　　　n. 化学制品/产品/物质/成分

【例句】The carbon dioxide would then be extracted and subjected to chemical reactions.

【译文】二氧化碳然后被提取出来，并将其进行化学反应。

chemist ['kemist]　　　　　　　*n*. 化学家，药剂师

【例句】As chemists，we are fascinated by computer sciences or molecular genetics.

【译文】作为化学家，我们对计算机科学或分子遗传学十分着迷。

chemotherapy [ˌkiːmə(u)'θerəpi]　　　　*n*. 化疗

【例句】His disease has already been diagnosed and treated with surgery, chemotherapy or radiation.

【译文】他的病已经确诊，并通过手术、化疗或放疗进行治疗。

cigar [si'gɑː]　　　　　　　　　　*n*. 雪茄烟

circular ['səːkjulə]　　　　　　*a*. 圆形的；循环的

circumstance [ˈsəːkəmstəns]

n. (pl.) 情形，环境；条件

【搭配】under the circumstances 在这种情况下，情况既然如此；under/in no circumstances 在任何情况下都不（放在句首要倒装）

【导学】辨析 circumstances，environment，setting，surroundings：circumstances 指某事或某动作发生时的情况，形势；environment 指周围的状况或条件，可以是自然环境，也可以是社会环境，可以是物质上的，也可以是精神上的；setting 指某一情形的背景或环境；surroundings 围绕物，周围的事物。

【例句】More importance should be attached to the child's life circumstances.

【译文】我们应该更加关注孩子的生存环境。

Day 6

transaction [trænˈzækʃən] n. 交易，事务，处理事务

【搭配】conduct transaction 进行交易

【例句】As they bought and sold assets, they had trouble remembering that each transaction could impact their monthly cash flow.

【译文】当他们买卖资产时，总是难以记住每笔交易都会对他们的每月现金流量产生影响。

transcend [træn'send]　　　　　　　*vt*. 超出，超越
　　　　　　　　　　　　　　（经验、理性、信念等的）范围

【导学】近义词：exceed，overreach，overrun，over-
　　　step，surpass，excess

【例句】She could never transcend her resentments
　　　against her mother's partiality for her
　　　brother.

【译文】母亲对弟弟的偏心使她心生怨恨，无法释怀。

transfer [træns'fə:] *vt*. 迁移，调动；换车；转让，过户
　　　　　　['trænsfə(r)] *n*. 迁移，调动；换车；转让，过户

【搭配】transfer sth. from...to 转移，调任，换乘

【例句】Transfer research results into commodities ac-
　　　cording to market rules.

【译文】将研究成果按市场规律转换成商品。

transform [træns'fɔ:m] *vt*. 转换，变形；变化，变压

【联想】change...into，turn...into 由……变成

【例句】Big challenges still await companies transfor-
　　　ming carbon dioxide to petrol.

【译文】巨大的挑战仍然横亘在公司将二氧化碳转化成
　　　汽油的道路上。

transistor [træn'zistə]　　　　　　*n*. 晶体管（收音机）

transit ['trænsit]　　　　　　　　　*n*. 通行，运输

【例句】 We observed the transit of Venus across the sun last night.

【译文】 我们昨晚观测到金星凌日。

transition [træn'ziʃən] *n*. 转变，变迁，过渡（时期）

【导学】 近义词：shift, passage, flux, passing, development, transformation, turn

【例句】 The transition from childhood to adulthood is always a critical time for everybody.

【译文】 从童年到成年的过渡对每个人来说都是一个关键的时期。

transplant [træns'plɑːnt] *vt*. 移栽，移种（植物等）；移植（器官）；使迁移，使移居

[' trænsplɑːnt] *n*. （器官的）移植

Day 6

【导学】 注意该词的名词形式同样也可以做定语。

【例句】 When any non-human organ is transplanted into a person, the body immediately recognizes it as foreign.

【译文】 当任何非人类的器官移植到人体内，身体很快便能识别出它是异物。

translation [træns'leiʃən] *n*. 翻译

transmit [trænz'mit] *vt*. 传送，传输，传达，传导，发射 *vi*. 发射信号，发报

【联想】 transmission *n*. 传输，传达

【搭配】 transmit a match live 实况转播比赛

【例句】 Most colds are acquired by children in school and then transmitted to adults.

【译文】 大多数感冒是孩子在学校得的，然后传染给了成年人。

transparent [træns'pεərənt]　　　　　*a*. 透明的

【联想】 transparency *n*. 透明度

【例句】 What we need is to start asking suppliers to be transparent about where and how their products are manufactured.

【译文】 我们要做的是开始要求供应商对其产品的生产地和生产流程保持透明公开。

transport ['trænspɔːt]　　　　　　　　*n*. 运输，运送
　　　　　[træns'pɔːt]　　　　　　　*vt*. 运输，运送

【联想】 transportation *n*. 运输，运输系统

【例句】 Additional social stresses may also occur because of the population explosion or problems arising from mass migration movements—themselves made relatively easy nowadays by modern means of transport.

【译文】 由于人口猛增或大量人口流变动（现在交通运输工具使大量人口流动变得相对容易）所引起

的各种社会问题也会对社会造成新的压力。

treatment [ˈtriːtmənt]　　*n*. 待遇，对待；治疗，疗法

trial [ˈtraɪəl]　　　　　　　　　*n*. 试验；审判

【搭配】be on trial 在试验中；在受审

【例句】Large trials are underway around the world to evaluate the idea.

【译文】全世界正在进行大规模试验来评估这个想法。

typical [ˈtɪpɪkəl]　　　　　*a*. 典型的，有代表性的；独有的，独特的

【搭配】be typical of 代表性的，典型的

【例句】A dormitory is the typical dwelling of a college student.

【译文】宿舍是大学生的典型住所。

Day 7

civil ['sivl]   *a.* 市民的，公民的，国民的；民间的；民事的，根据民法的；文职的

【例句】He left the army and resumed civil life.

【译文】他离开了军队，恢复了平民生活。

civilian [si'viljən]   *a.* 平民的，民用的，民众的

civilization [ˌsivilai'zeiʃən]   *n.* 文明，文化

【联想】civilize *vt.* 使开化，使文明，教化

【例句】Both civilization and culture are fairly modern words, having come into use during the 19th century by anthropologists.

【译文】文明和文化都是相当时髦的词汇，是人类学家在 19 世纪开始使用的词汇。

claim [kleim] *n.* （根据权利提出）要求，要求权，主张，要求而得到的东西 *vt.* （根据权利）要求，认领，声称，主张，需要

【导学】辨析 claim，proclaim：claim 一般指声称对某物的拥有权；proclaim 常为官方正式宣布。

【例句】 At present, it is too easy to make unverified claims.

【译文】 目前，提出未经证实的观点太容易了。

classic ['klæsik]　　　　　　　　*a*. 经典的；第一流的
　　　　　　　　　　　　　　　　　　n. 杰作，名著

【导学】 辨析 classic, classical：classic 的意思是 "经典的"，描述能经受历史考验的物品；classical "古典的"，与 modern 相对。

【例句】 The classic sleepwalker is Shakespeare's Lady Macbeth.

【译文】 经典的梦游者是莎士比亚笔下的麦克白夫人。

classify ['klæsifai]　　　　　　　　*vt*. 分类，分级

【联想】 classification *n*. 分类，分级

【例句】 Stereotypes seem unavoidable, given the way the human mind seeks to categorize and classify information.

【译文】 鉴于人类大脑进行信息的归类和分类的方法，刻板印象似乎是不可避免的。

climate ['klaimit]　　　　　　　　*n*. 气候；风气，思潮

【联想】 climatic *a*. 气候的，与气候有关的

【例句】 Models will never provide a straightforward prediction of how the climate will change.

【译文】 模型永远无法直接预测气候如何变化。

clinic ['klinik]　　　　*n*. 诊所；（医院的）门诊部；
　　　　　　　　　　　门诊时间；会诊时间；私人诊所；
　　　　　　　　　　　专科医院；门诊治疗部；临床实习

【联想】 clinical *a*. 临床的；clinically *ad*. 临床地

【例句】 The centre is unattached to any hospital or clinic.

【译文】 这个中心不附属于任何医院或诊所。

collaborate [kə'læbəreit]　　　　*v*. 合作，协作

【联想】 collaboration *n*. 合作，协作

【例句】 Biologists and sociologists will have to start treating one other with a new respect and learn how to collaborate outside their comfort zones.

【译文】 生物学家和社会学家将不得不以一种新的尊重来对待彼此，并学习如何在自己的舒适区之外进行合作。

colleague ['kɔli:g]　　　　*n*. 同事，同僚

【导学】 辨析 colleague, partner：colleague 指同事、同行、职员或学院教工的同僚之一；partner 指伙伴，同伙，或在一项活动或一个涉及共同利益的领域内与另一人或其他人联合或有联系的人，尤指企业合作人、配偶、舞伴、

搭档等。

【例句】 Gould and her colleagues suspect that learning itself might bolster the new neurons' survival.

【译文】 古尔德和她的同事怀疑，学习本身可能会促进新神经元存活。

combine [kəmˈbain]　　　　　　v. 结合，联合，化合

【搭配】 combine with 与……联合（化合、结合）

【联想】 combination n. 结合，联合

【例句】 Psycho therapy, specifically problem-behavioral therapy needs to be combined.

【译文】 心理疗法，尤其是问题行为疗法，应该结合起来。

comment [ˈkɔment]　　　　　　n. /v. 解说，评论

【搭配】 comment on/upon 评论，谈论，对……提意见

【例句】 The range of news is from local crime to international politics, from sport to business to fashion to science, and the range of comment and special features as well, from editorial pages to feature articles and interviews to criticisms of books, art, theatre and music.

【译文】 新闻的范围从当地的犯罪到国际政治，从体育到商业，到时尚，到科学。评论和特写的范围

也是从社论到专栏文章，以及对书籍、艺术、戏剧和音乐的评论。

commerce [ˈkɔmə(ː)s]　　　　　　*n*. 商业，贸易

【联想】commercial *a*. 商业的，商务的 *n*. 商业广告

【例句】Commercial companies produce false neoantigens for the sake of competition.

【译文】为了竞争，商业公司不惜生产假的新抗原。

communicate [kəˈmjuːnikeit]　 *vi*. 沟通；传达，传播
　　　　　　　　　　　　　　　vt. 传达；交流；通信

【搭配】communicate with 和……联系，和……通信
　　　　communicate sth. to sb. 把……传达给某人

【联想】communication *n*. 通讯；通信；交际，交流；传达，传送

【例句】Unless the families can communicate with caregivers, they cannot begin to trust them.

【译文】除非能够与照护者沟通，否则家庭成员无法开始信任他们。

community [kəˈmjuːniti]　　　　　　　　*n*. 社区

【例句】A hero has a story of adventure to tell and community will listen to.

【译文】英雄总有冒险的故事可讲，而公众又愿意去听。

comparable [ˈkɔmpərəbl]　　*a*. 可比较的，比得上的

【搭配】be comparable with 可与……相比的，与……
类似的；be comparable to 可与……比拟的，
与……匹敌的

【例句】Nevertheless, children in both double-income
and "male breadwinner" households spent
comparable amount of time interacting with
their parents.

【译文】然而，在双收入家庭和父亲为收入来源的家庭
中，孩子和父母互动的时间相当。

comparative [kəm'pærətiv]   *a*. 比较的，相当的

comparison [kəm'pærisn]   *n*. 比较；对比

【搭配】in comparison with 与……比较
by comparison 比较起来

【例句】The comparison is generally made between
children and adults.

【译文】这种比较通常是在儿童和成人之间进行的。

compassionate [kəm'pæʃənit]   *a*. 有同情心的，
深表同情的

【联想】compassion *n*. 同情

【例句】In the office, she had found her physician
compassionate and warm.

【译文】在办公室里，她发现她的医生们富有同情心和
热情。

compensate ['kɔmpənseit]　　　　*vt*. 补偿，偿还，酬报（for）；给……付工钱；赔偿

【搭配】compensate sb. for 因……而赔偿某人
　　　　compensate for 弥补

【联想】compensatory *a*. 补偿性的，弥补性的

【例句】To compensate for his unpleasant experiences he drank a little more than how much was good for him.

【译文】为了借酒消愁，他喝得有点过了头。

compensation [kɔmpen'seiʃən]　　　　*n*. 补偿，赔偿

【导学】该词属于常考词汇，经常出现在阅读和词汇部分。

【例句】The insurance company paid him ＄10,000 in compensation after his accident.

【译文】事故之后，保险公司支付给他一万美元作为赔偿。

complain [kəm'plein]　　　　*vi*. 抱怨，诉苦，申诉

【搭配】complain to sb. of/about sth. 向某人抱怨某事
　　　　complain of doing sth. 抱怨做某事

【联想】complaint *n*. 抱怨，怨言；控告

【导学】complain 后面只接 that 从句做宾语，不直接跟 sb. 或 sth. 做宾语。

【例句】Technically, insomnia is defined as a "complaint", and since animals can't complain, it's difficult to measure in them.

【译文】严格说来，失眠被定义为"抱怨"，因为动物不能抱怨，所以很难对它们进行测量。

complement ['kɔmplimənt]   *n.* 补足；余数；补语

【联想】complementary *a.* 补足的，补充的

【例句】Movie directors use music to complement the action on the screen.

【译文】电影导演运用音乐与屏幕上的情节相配合。

complicated ['kɔmplikeitid]   *a.* 错综复杂的，难懂的

【联想】complicate *vt.* 使复杂化，使混乱，使难懂

【例句】This is too complicated a matter to settle all by myself.

【译文】这事太复杂，我一人难以对付。

complication [ˌkɔmpli'keiʃ(ə)n]   *n.* 错杂，新增的困难，新出现的问题；并发症

【例句】His broken arm healed well, but he died of pneumonia which followed as a complication.

【译文】他的断臂愈合得很好，但最终死于肺炎这一并发症。

conceal [kən'si:l]   *vt.* 隐瞒，隐藏，隐蔽

【搭配】conceal sth. from sb. 对某人隐瞒某事物

【例句】 John's mindless exterior concealed a warm and kindhearted nature.

【译文】 约翰漫不经心的外表掩盖了他热情、善良的本性。

concentrate ['kɔnsentreit]   *vt*. 集中；聚集；浓缩
  vi. 集中，专心

【搭配】 concentrate on/upon 集中在，专心于

【联想】 concentration *n*. 专注，专心；集中；浓度

【例句】 Among many other issues, this rapid concentration makes cities a front line in the battles against climate change and pollution.

【译文】 在许多其他问题中，这种快速集中使城市成为对抗气候变化和污染的前线。

safeguard ['seifgɑːd]   *v*. 保护，保障，捍卫
  n. 安全设施，保护措施

【例句】 It is deemed necessary to protect the entire population through vaccination, so as to safeguard lives.

【译文】 人们认为有必要通过接种疫苗来保护整个人口，以保护生命。

sake [seik]   *n*. 缘故，理由

【搭配】 for the sake of 为了

【例句】 We should continue to integrate theory with

practice, study for the sake of application, and acquire a better understanding of the theory of Marxism.

【译文】我们要继续理论联系实际，学以致用，提高马克思主义的理论水平。

satellite ['sætəlait]   *n.* 卫星，人造卫星

【搭配】launch a satellite 发射卫星

【例句】We receive television pictures by satellite.

【译文】我们通过人造卫星接收电视图像。

satisfactory [ˌsætis'fæktəri]   *a.* 令人满意的

【例句】The plan is almost satisfactory in every way.

【译文】这个计划几近完美。

saving ['seiviŋ]   *n.* 储蓄；(*pl.*) 储蓄金，存款

【搭配】deposit one's savings 存款

scale [skeil]   *n.* 标度，刻度 (*pl.*) 天平，天平盘；标尺，比例尺；音阶

【搭配】on a large scale 大规模地

【例句】It may be possible for large-scale change to occur without leaders with magnetic personalities, but the pace of change would be slow.

【译文】缺乏独特个人魅力的领导者也有可能推动大规

模的变革，但变化的进度可能会慢一些。

scan [skæn]   *v.* /*n.* 浏览；扫描

【例句】He scanned *Time* magazine while waiting at the doctor's office.

【译文】在医生的办公室候诊时，他翻阅了《时代》周刊。

scarcely ['skɛəsli]   *ad.* 几乎不；勉强

【搭配】scarcely... when 一……就

【联想】scarce *a.* 稀少的，罕见的

【例句】It is scarcely practical for seriously ill people.

【译文】这对重病患者几乎不实用。

scare [skɛə]   *vt.* 惊吓，使恐惧 *vi.* 惊慌，惊恐

【例句】A lot of people felt the same way, but were too scared to say anything.

【译文】很多人都有同样的感觉，但都怕得什么也不敢说。

scatter ['skætə]   *vi.* 撒，驱散，散开；散布，散播 *vt.* 分散，消散

【导学】辨析 scatter, disperse, spread：scatter 指由于外力使人或物杂乱地向不同的方向散开或散播；disperse 指有目的地、安全地解散或彻底散开，范围较前者广；spread 指在表层分

散，也可指疾病、谣言的传播。

【例句】 I hate to scold，but you mustn't scatter your things all over the place.

【译文】 我不想训斥你，但你不该总把东西到处乱丢。

scenario [sə'nɑːriəʊ]　　*n*. 脚本；方案；设想；预测；
　　　　　　　　　　　　　　（电影或戏剧的）剧情梗概

【例句】 Let me suggest a possible scenario.

【译文】 我来设想一种可能出现的情况。

scratch [skrætʃ]　　*v*. 搔，抓，扒；勾销，删除
　　　　　　　　　　　　　n. 搔，抓，抓痕

【搭配】 scratch a living 勉强维持生活

【例句】 The scratch on your hand will soon be well.

【译文】 你手上的划伤不久就会好。

scream [skriːm]　　　　　　　　　*vi*. 尖叫

【例句】 All children spent more time looking at the eyes of a face that was paired with the loud scream than the face that was not paired with the scream.

【译文】 所有的孩子都花更多时间注视与尖叫声配对的脸的眼睛，而不是那些没有与尖叫声配对的面孔。

segregate ['segrigeit]　　　*v*. 隔离并区别对待
　　　　　　　　（不同种族、宗教或性别的人）；（使）隔离

【联想】segregation *n*. 种族隔离；隔离

shallow [ˈʃæləʊ] *a*. 浅的；浅薄的，肤浅的
                      n. (*pl*.) 浅滩，浅处

【例句】Too much texting can make you shallow.

【译文】发太多文字信息会让人变得肤浅。

shortly [ˈʃɔːtli] *ad*. 立刻，马上

【例句】A young girl suffering from an advanced stage of rabies died shortly after the injection procedure had commenced.

【译文】一名患有狂犬病晚期的年轻女孩在注射疗程开始后不久就去世了。

shrink [ʃriŋk] *vi*. 起皱，收缩；退缩，畏缩

【例句】Shrinking landfill space, and rising costs for burying and burning rubbish are forcing local governments to look more closely at recycling.

【译文】掩埋式垃圾处理场可占用的空间逐渐缩小，同时，掩埋和燃烧垃圾的成本却在增长，这迫使当地政府更加重视回收利用。

signal [ˈsignl] *n*. 信号，暗号 *v*. 发信号，打暗号

【联想】signature *n*. 签字，签名

【例句】They all seemed to be plagued by annoying technical issues: a weak Wi-Fi signal, dropped connections，wrong phone numbers in the chart.

【译文】他们似乎都受到了恼人的技术问题的困扰：Wi-Fi信号弱、连接中断、图表中的电话号码错误等。

significant [sig'nifikənt]   *a*. 重大的；重要的；意味深长的

【联想】significance *n*. 意义，含义；重要性

【例句】A significant proportion of these products are made in the developing world by low-paid people with inadequate labor rights.

【译文】这些产品中的很大一部分是由低收入、劳动权利不足的人在发展中国家制造的。

simulate ['simjuleit]   *vt*. 模仿，模拟；假装，冒充

【例句】We used to use this trick in the army to simulate illness.

【译文】我们在军队服役时常用这一伎俩装病。

situated ['sitjueitid]   *a*. 位于，坐落于

【搭配】be situated at/in/on 位于

【例句】The housing development must be situated near public transportation.

【译文】住房开发必须位于靠近公共交通的地方。

Day 7

skeptical [ˈskeptikəl]　　　　　　　a. 表示怀疑的

【导学】 和它的近义词一起记忆：doubtable,
suspicious。

【例句】 Ignorant people were skeptical of Columbus'
theory that the earth is round.

【译文】 那时，无知的人对于哥伦布的地球是圆形的理
论表示怀疑。

slaughter [ˈslɔːtə]　　　　　n. 屠杀，杀戮；屠宰

【导学】 表示"杀"的词还有：butcher 屠宰，屠杀；
massacre 残杀，集体屠杀；carnage（尤指在
战场上的）残杀，大屠杀，流血；assassinate
暗杀，行刺。

【例句】 I could not stand to watch them slaughter the
cattle.

【译文】 看到他们在屠杀那群牛，我受不了。

soak [səuk]　　　　　　　　　　v. 浸湿，浸透

【例句】 Others thought that the oceans would soak up
any extra CO_2.

【译文】 其他人认为海洋会吸收任何额外的二氧化碳。

soar [sɔː, soə]　　　　vi. 高飞，翱翔；高涨，猛增

【例句】 With soaring healthcare cost and long waits
for medical procedures，it is becoming in-

creasingly difficult to find quality，affordable treatment.

【译文】随着医疗费用的飙升和医疗程序的漫长等待，越来越难找到高质量、负担得起的治疗方法。

social ['səʊʃəl]　　　　*a*. 社会的；社交的，交际的

【例句】Social studies is the study of how man lives in societies.

【译文】社科课程是研究人们怎样在社会中生活的学科。

solar ['səʊlə]　　　　*a*. 太阳的，日光的

【搭配】solar system 太阳系

【例句】The best bet might be to invest heavily in improving solar technology and energy storage.

【译文】最好的办法可能是大力投资于改进太阳能技术和能源储存效率。

sophisticated [sə'fistikeitid]　　*a*. 先进的，复杂的；精密的；老于世故的

【例句】The British in particular are becoming more sophisticated and creative.

【译文】特别是英国人变得更加成熟和有创造力。

specialist ['speʃəlist]　　　　　　*n*. 专家

【搭配】a specialist in/on 在……方面的专家

specialize [ˈspeʃəlaiz]　　　　*vi.* 专攻，专门研究

【搭配】specialize in 专攻

【例句】Humans have specialized decision systems in addition to generalized reasoning ability.

【译文】除一般推理能力外，人类还具有特殊决策能力。

species [ˈspiːʃiːz]　　　　*n.* (物)种，种类

【例句】Humans are the only species known to have consciousness.

【译文】人类是唯一具有意识的物种。

specific [spiˈsifik]　　　　*n.* 特效药；(*pl.*) 细节
　　　　　　　　　　a. 详细而精确的，明确的；特殊的，
　　　　　　　　　　特效的；(生物)种的

【联想】specifically *ad.* 特定地，明确地

【例句】Our exceptional brainpower arose through evolutionary pressures to acquire specific cognitive skills.

【译文】我们非凡的智能是通过获得特定认知技能的进化压力产生的。

Day 8

confidence [ˈkɔnfidəns]　　　　*n*. 信任，信心；秘密

【搭配】in confidence 秘密地；with confidence 充满
　　　　自信地；have confidence in 对……有信心

confident [ˈkɔnfidənt]　　　　　*a*. 确信的，有自信的

【搭配】be/feel confident in/of 确信某事

【联想】be/feel certain of，be/feel sure of，be convinced
　　　　of，have confidence in 确信某事

【例句】He is confident that scientists can block trans-
　　　　mission of malaria to humans.

【译文】他确信科学家能够阻止疟疾向人类的传播。

confidential [ˌkɔnfiˈdenʃəl]　　　*a*. 秘密的，机密的；
　　　　　　　　　　　　　　　　　　表示信任（或亲密）的

【例句】All information reported to the commission is
　　　　considered confidential.

【译文】所有汇报给委员会的信息都被定为机密。

confirmation [ˌkɔnfəˈmeiʃən]　　　*n*. 确定，确立，
　　　　　　　　　　　　　　　　　证实；确认，批准

【联想】confirm *vt*. 证实，进一步确定，确认；批准

【例句】 Wainwright found confirmation that Morrell gave Hitler antibiotics as a precaution in a recent translation of Morrell's own diary.

【译文】 温顿特最近在翻译莫雷尔的私人日记时确认，莫雷尔给希特勒注射了抗生素预防针。

confront [kən'frʌnt]   *vt.* 使面对，使遭遇

【联想】 confrontation *n.* 面对；对峙（抗）；对质

【例句】 It makes people differ from each other confronting the same nutrients.

【译文】 这使人们面对相同的营养素时彼此（反应）不同。

conserve [kən'sə:v]   *vt.* 保存，保护；节约，节省

【导学】 conserve，protect，reserve，preserve：conserve 指保护从而使其不受损失或伤害，也指节约，谨慎或省俭地使用，避免浪费；protect 指保护使免于受到损坏、攻击、偷盗或伤害；reserve 指收藏保留，如用于将来使用或某个特殊的目的，也指"预订，预约"；preserve 意为"保存，保持，收藏"，指保护某物不受破坏，使之完好无损。

【例句】 If no one owns the resource concerned, no one has an interest in conserving it or fostering it：fish is the best example of this.

【译文】如果相关的资源没有主人，就不会有人有兴趣去保存或培养它；鱼就是这方面的最好例证。

considerable [kən'sidərəbl]   *a*. 相当的；可观的

【例句】The advantages of these outside interests and positions have been considerable for individuals.

【译文】这些外部利益和职位给个人带来的优势是相当可观的。

considerate [kən'sidərit]   *a*. 考虑周到的，体谅的，体贴的

【联想】consideration *n*. 考虑
【搭配】take... into consideration 纳入考虑范围
【例句】She is always considerate of my feelings.
【译文】她总是很考虑我的感受。

consolidate [kən'sɔlideit]   *v*. 加固，巩固

【导学】该词属于常考词汇，尤其出现在词汇部分。考生要注意常用的相关同义词：solidify（使……凝固，使……团结，巩固），strengthen（加强，巩固），unify（使联合，统一）。

【例句】Consolidate and develop socialist relations characterized by equality，unity and mutual assistance among all ethnic groups for common prosperity and progress.

【译文】巩固和发展平等、团结、互助的社会主义民族关系，实现各民族共同繁荣和进步。

constant [ˈkɔnstənt]　　　　*a.* 不断的，持续的；始终如一的；坚定的，忠实的；恒定的，经常的

【导学】辨析 constant，continual，continuous：constant 表示连续发生的，在性质、价值或范围上持久不变的，始终如一的；continual 表示有规律地或经常地发生，强调中间有间断的连续；continuous 表示不间断的连续。

【例句】The newly-designed machine can help the room maintain a constant and steady temperature.

【译文】这种新设计的机器能够使房间保持一个稳定不变的温度。

consult [kənˈsʌlt]　　*vt.* 请教，咨询；查阅；就诊
　　　　　　　　　　　　　　vi. 商量；会诊

【联想】consultation *n.* 咨询

【搭配】consult…about…向……讨教某事；consult with…about…跟某人商量某事

【导学】辨析 consult，consult with：consult 指"向……请教或咨询"，或指"参考，查阅"；consult with 指"磋商，交换意见"。

【例句】Many generalists will consult with specialists on complicated cases.（2011）

【译文】很多全科医生都会在复杂的案例上咨询专科医生。

consultant [kən'sʌltənt]　　　　　　　　*n.* 顾问

【导学】辨析 consultant，guide：consultant 指提供专家意见或专业意见的人；guide 指在方法或道路上引导或指导另一人的人，或在行为等方面堪称他人楷模的人。

【例句】I think we need to see all investment consultants before we make an expensive mistake.

【译文】我认为我们必须拜访所有的投资顾问以免犯下代价昂贵的错误。

contact ['kɒntækt]　　　　　*n.* /*vt.* 接触，联系，交往

【联想】container *n.* 容器，集装箱

【搭配】be in (out of) contact with 与……有（失去）联系
keep in touch with sb. 与某人保持联系

【例句】Others realize it when they contact biological half-siblings who have the same disorder.

【译文】其他人在接触患有同样疾病的同父异母兄弟姐妹时意识到了这一点。

contaminate [kən'tæmineit]　　　　*vt.* 弄脏，污染

【例句】Now a paper in *Science* argues that organic chemicals in the rock come mostly from con-

Day 8

tamination on earth rather than bacteria on Mars.

【译文】 最近《科学》上的一篇文章宣称：岩石中的有机化学物质主要来自地球本身的污染，而并非来自火星上的细菌。

---

contract ['kɔntrækt]　　　　*n*. 契约，合同，包工
　　　　　[kən'trækt]　　　　*v*. 收缩；感染；订约

【搭配】 enter into/make a contract（with sb.）（for sth.）（与某人）（为事）订立合约；sign a contract 签订合同；contract with 与……订合同

---

contrast ['kɔntræst]　　　　　　*v. /n*. 对比，对照

【搭配】 in contrast with/to 和……形成对比（对照）contrast A with B 把 A 与 B 对照

【例句】 The ability, called contrast sensitivity function, allows people to discern even subtle changes.

【译文】 这种能力被称为对比敏感度功能，可以让人们分辨出十分细微的变化。

---

controversial [ˌkɔntrə'vəːʃəl]　　　　*a*. 争论的；引起争论的；被议论的；可疑的

【例句】 Many members of the medical community

prefer to avoid becoming involved in controversial issues.

【译文】医学界的许多成员倾向于避免卷入有争议的问题。

convention [kən'venʃən]   n. 习俗，惯例；
大会，会议；公约

【联想】conventional a. 普通的，常见的；习惯的，常规的

【搭配】break established conventions 打破成规；sign a convention of peace with a neighbouring country 与邻国签订一项和平协定

【例句】Such buildings are often cheaper than those built using conventional methods.

【译文】这样的建筑通常比使用传统材料的成本低廉。

cooperate [kəu'ɔpəreit]   vi. 合作，协作，相配合

【搭配】cooperate with sb. in doing sth. 与某人合作做某事

【例句】The British cooperated with the French in building the new craft.

【译文】英、法两国合作制造这种新式飞船。

coordinate [kəu'ɔ:dinit]   v. (使) 协调，调整；
(使) 互相配合

【搭配】coordinate with each other 互相配合

【例句】 What steps do you take, and how do you coordinate care?

【译文】 您采取了哪些步骤，如何协调护理？

corporate ['kɔːpərit]　　a. 公司的；法人组织的；社会团体的；共同的；自治的

【联想】 corporation n. 公司，团体

【例句】 Organizations are becoming more corporate and less enlightened.

【译文】 组织正变得越来越企业化，也越来越不开明。

counter ['kauntə]　　n. 计算器，计数器，计算者；柜台；筹码 ad. / a. 相反地（的）

【联想】 over-the-counter（OTC）非处方药

【例句】 Take one of the over-the-counter decongestant, and maybe a couple of Aspirins.

【译文】 服用一种非处方减充血剂，也可以吃几片阿司匹林。

counterpart ['kauntəpɑːt]　　n. 对等的人；副本

【导学】 该词属于常考词汇，主要出现在词汇选择和阅读部分。其中 counter 原指"柜台"，可想象成顾客和服务生面对面的场景，转义为"相对的"。

【例句】 Your right hand is the counterpart of your

left hand.

【译文】你的右手是你左手的相对物。

crash [kræʃ]   *v. / n.* 摔坏，坠毁

【导学】辨析 crash，crush，smash：crash 指 "坠毁"，碰撞中造成的突然毁损；crush 指 "压碎"，把（石头或矿石等）挤压、捣碎或碾成小碎块或粉末；smash 指 "打碎"，或突然地、大声地、猛力地把某种东西毁成碎片。

【例句】Smaller crash-test dummies have also been used to represent children inside crashing cars.

【译文】较小的碰撞测试假人也被用来代表碰撞汽车内的儿童。

create [kri'eit] *vt.* 创造，创作；产生；制造，建立

【联想】creative *a.* 有创造力的，创造性的

【例句】I created the Obituary Writing Program at Georgetown University during my first year of medical school.

【译文】在医学院的第一年，我在乔治城大学开设了讣告写作课程。

credential [krə'denʃl]   *n.* 资质
                                             vt. 提供证明书（或证件）

【例句】In many cases, green credentials promote

green economy.

【译文】很多情况下，绿色资质会促进绿色经济。

---

crime [kraim]　　　　　　　　　*n.* 罪，罪行，犯罪

【联想】criminal *a.* 犯罪的，刑事的　*n.* 罪犯，刑事犯

【例句】Most crime goes unreported so it is hard to pick out trends from the data.

【译文】大多数犯罪都没有被报道，因此很难从数据中找出趋势。

---

criterion [krai'tiəriən]　　　　　　　*n.* 标准，准则

【导学】该词经常用于指代各类赛事的评分标准，常见的近义词：rule（准则），standard（标准），regulation（规则）等。

【例句】The most important criterion for assessment in this contest is originality of design.

【译文】这次比赛最重要的评判标准就是设计的原创性。

---

critical ['kritikəl]　　　　　　*a.* 批评的，批判的；
　　　　　　　　　　　　　　　　　　危急的，紧要的

【搭配】be critical of 挑剔，不满

【例句】We are at a critical point in our nation's history.

【译文】我们现在正处于我们国家历史中的一个关键时刻。

criticize ['kritisaiz]　　　　　　*vt*. 批评，评论

【联想】 criticism *n*. 批评，评论；critic *n*. 评论家

【例句】 The purpose of the author is to comment and
criticize.

【译文】 作者写作的目的是为了评论和谴责。

crucial ['kruːʃiəl, 'kruːʃəl]　　　*a*. 关键的，决定性的

【例句】 During this crucial period of health system
reform，we've been advocating for strategies
that support preventive medicine.

【译文】 在这个卫生系统改革的关键时期，我们一直在
倡导支持预防医学的战略。

cultivate ['kʌltiveit]　　　　　*vt*. 耕作，栽培，养殖；
　　　　　　　　　　　　　　　　　培养，陶冶，发展

【例句】 They have enough money and leisure time to
cultivate an interest in the arts.

【译文】 他们有足够的金钱和空闲时间来培养艺术方面
的兴趣。

culture ['kʌltʃə]　　　　　　*n*. 文化，文明；教养

【例句】 They experience culture shock.

【译文】 他们经历了文化冲突。

speculate ['spekjuleit]　　　　　*vi.* 思索，推测；投机

【搭配】speculate about/on/over 推测；speculate in 投机

【例句】We are living in the here and can only speculate about the hereafter.

【译文】我们生活在现在，只能预测未来。

spiritual ['spiritjuəl]　　　　*a.* 精神（上）的，心灵的

stable ['steibl]　　　　　　　　*a.* 安定的，稳定的

【联想】stabilize *vt.* 使稳定，使稳固

【例句】People guess that the price of oil should remain stable for the rest of the year.

【译文】人们估计在今年剩下的日子里油价会保持稳定。

statement ['steitmənt]　　　　　　*n.* 陈述，声明

【搭配】confirm a statement 证实某一说法

statistic [stə'tistik]　　　　　　　*n.* 统计数值

【例句】Even reliable sets of statistics can be difficult to compare.

【译文】即使是可靠的统计数据都很难对比。

status ['steitəs]　　*n.* 地位，身份；情形，状况

【例句】China believes that nuclear-weapon states should respect the status of nuclear-weapon-free zones and assume corresponding obligations.

【译文】中国认为，核武器国家应尊重无核武器区的地位并承担相应的义务。

steady ['stedi]　　　　　*a*. 稳定，不变；稳固，平稳；坚定，扎实 *v*. （使）稳定

【例句】We on the staff took personal pride and delight in his steady progress.

【译文】我们作为员工为他稳定的进步感到骄傲和高兴。

stimulate ['stimjuleit]　　　*vt*. 刺激，激励，使兴奋

【搭配】stimulate sb. into/to sth. 鼓励某人做

【例句】An important property of a scientific theory is its ability to stimulate further research and further thinking about a particular topic.

【译文】科学理论最重要的特性在于它针对某个特定主题能激发深入的研究和思考。

stimulus ['stimjuləs]　　　　　　　*n*. 刺激物

【导学】stimulus 后通常与介词 to 搭配。

【例句】During the first two months of a baby's life, the stimulus that produces a smile is a pair of eyes.

【译文】婴儿出生的头两个月，刺激他微笑的是别人的眼睛。

Day 8

strategy ['strætidʒi]   *n.* 战略；策略

【搭配】adopt/apply/pursue a strategy 采取策略

【例句】Meanwhile, we will also carry out the open strategy of Going Global and encourage qualified companies with competence to make overseas investment.

【译文】同时，我们还要实施"走出去"开放战略，鼓励有条件有实力的企业到境外投资办厂。

substance ['sʌbstəns]   *n.* 物质；实质，本质；要旨，大意

【搭配】in substance 大体上是，从本质上说

【例句】Water consists of various chemical substance.

【译文】水由各种不同的化学物质构成。

subtract [səb'trækt]   *vt.* 减，减去

【例句】He could add and subtract, but hadn't learned to divide.

【译文】他会做加减法，但还没有学会除法。

suicide ['sjuisaid]   *n.* 自杀

【搭配】commit suicide 自杀

【例句】Suicide is a very real risk for young people who suffer from clinical depression.

【译文】对于患有临床抑郁症的年轻人来说，自杀是一个真实存在的风险。

superficial [ˌsjuːpəˈfɪʃəl] *a*. 表面的；肤浅的，浅薄的

【例句】 Because we teach you to improve your ability to think critically，to analyze situations，not just superficially.

【译文】 因为我们教你提高自己批判性思维的能力和分析情况的能力，而不仅仅是表面上的。

surgery [ˈsəːdʒəri] *n*. 外科，外科手术

【联想】 surgical *a*. 外科（医术）的；外科用的，外科手术的

【例句】 What they say during surgery may distress the patient afterwards.

【译文】 他们在手术过程中所说的话可能会使患者在术后感到压抑。

surveillance [səˈveiləns] *n*. 监控；（对犯罪嫌疑人或可能发生犯罪的地方的）监视

【例句】 His condition can be kept under continuous surveillance at home.

【译文】 他的病情可以在家中得到持续监测。

sustain [səsˈtein] *vt*. 支撑，撑住；经受，忍耐

【联想】 sustainable *a*. 可以忍受的，足可支撑的，养得起的

【例句】 But diets that restrict certain food groups are difficult or unhealthy to sustain over time.

【译文】 但是限制某些食物种类的饮食很难长时间维持，或者说长时间坚持会不利于健康。

sympathetic [ˌsimpəˈθetik]　　　 *a*. 同情的，共鸣的

【搭配】 be sympathetic to... 对……表示同情

【联想】 sympathize *vt*. 同情，怜悯，共鸣
sympathy *n*. 同情，同情心；赞同，同感
sympathize with sb., show sympathy towards sb., feel/express sympathy for/with sb., have sympathy for sb. 同情

symptom [ˈsimptəm]　　　　　　 *n*. 症状，征候

【搭配】 have/show the symptoms of a cold 有感冒的症状

【例句】 I didn't need any specific medical input or symptom control, although I was in a mess physically.

【译文】 我不需要任何具体的医疗输入或症状控制，尽管我的身体一团糟。

synthetic [sinˈθetik]　　 *a*. 合成的，人工的；综合的
　　　　　　　　　　　 n. 人工制品（尤指化学合成物）

【例句】 The store now offers 531 varieties of synthetic fabrics, all Chinese-made.

【译文】 这个店现在出售 531 种合成纤维，全部都是中国生产的。

Day *9*

dash [dæʃ]　　　　　　　　　 *vt*. 猛掷，猛撞 *vi*. 猛冲
　　　　　　　　　　　　　　 n. 猛冲，短跑；破折号

【例句】The boat was dashed against the rocks.

【译文】那船猛地撞到礁石上。

data [ˈdeitə]　　　　　 *n*. (datum 的复数) 资料，材料

【导学】做主语时，谓语可以是单数，也可以是复数。

【例句】There are more than 2.5 million workers who
　　　　need help, according to Labour Department
　　　　data.

【译文】根据劳动部的数据，有 250 多万名工人需要
　　　　帮助。

database [ˈdeitəbeis]　　　　　　　　 *n*. 数据库

【导学】该词在历年考题中均出现在阅读部分。需
　　　　要注意的是，data 来源于 datum，表达复
　　　　数概念。

【例句】This information is combined with a map
　　　　database.

【译文】这一信息同地图数据库有效地结合在一起。

deadline ['dedlain]　　　*n.* 最后期限，截止交稿日期

【例句】Last year Europe missed the deadline it had set itself in 2010 to eradicate measles.

【译文】去年，欧洲错过了 2010 年设定的消灭麻疹的最后期限。

deadly ['dedli]　　　*a.* 致命的，致死的；极有害的

【导学】辨析 deadly，fatal，mortal：deadly 意为"可能致死的"（likely to cause or able to produce death），表示能够或可能引起死亡，但不一定有导致死的结果；fatal 意为"导致死亡的"（causing or resulting in death），多指已经或将导致死亡，强调死亡是不可避免的；mortal 意为"死亡的"，指未能永存。

【例句】It was the worst tragedy in maritime history, six times more deadly than the Titanic.

【译文】这是航海史上一次空前的灾难，所造成的损失是泰坦尼克号的六倍之多。

debate [di'beit]　　　*vt.* 争论，辩论

【例句】We debated the advantages and disadvantages of filming famous works.

【译文】关于把名著拍成电影的优点和缺点，我们进行了辩论。

decade [ˈdekeid]   *n.* 十年

【例句】 For the past decade or so, practical courses, such as computer and business, have gained tremendous development on college campuses.

【译文】 过去十年来，实用性课程，诸如计算机和商业课程已在大学校园中得到极大的发展。

decay [diˈkei]   *v.* 腐烂；衰退 *n.* 衰退，腐烂

【例句】 Dr. Li of the U. S. Department of Agriculture, has found that oranges can be prevented from decaying by the use of certain chemicals containing sulfur compounds.

【译文】 美国农业部的李博士发现，使用某种含硫的化合物能防止橘子腐烂。

decrease [diːˈkriːs]   *v. / n.* 减少，减小

【例句】 Delaying treatment could lead to decreased heart function or even death.

【译文】 延误治疗可能会导致心脏功能衰退甚至死亡。

dedicate [ˈdedikeit]   *vt.* 奉献

【例句】 I want to see all of us dedicate ourselves to the principles for which we fought.

【译文】 我希望看到所有的人献身于我们为之奋斗的原则。

101

degrade [di'greid]　　　　　*v.* 分解，降级，使受屈辱

【例句】Insulin needs to be kept cold because it is made of weak chemical bonds that degrade at temperatures above 40 degrees Fahrenheit.

【译文】胰岛素需要冷藏，因为它由弱化学键组成，在40华氏度以上的温度下会降解。

deliberate [di'libəreit]　　　　　*a.* 故意的；深思熟虑的

v. 仔细考虑

【例句】Sometimes the messages are conveyed through deliberate, conscious gestures.

【译文】有时，信息是通过故意的、下意识的手势表达的。

delicate ['delikit]　　　　*a.* 纤弱的，娇嫩的，易碎的；优美的，精美的，精致的；微妙的，棘手的；灵敏的，精密的

【例句】Delicate plants must be protected from cold wind and frost.

【译文】娇弱的植物必须妥善保护，以避免风霜的侵袭。

democracy [di'mɔkrəsi]　　*n.* 民主，民主制；民主国家

【联想】democratic *a.* 民主的，有民主精神（作风）的

【例句】The author makes it a point to consider the consequences of compromising democracy.

【译文】作者认为有必要考虑损害民主的后果。

demonstrate ['demənstreit]　　*vt*. 表明；论证；演示
　　　　　　　　　　　　　　　　　vi. 示威

【搭配】demonstrate against 示威反对
【例句】History has demonstrated that countries with different social systems can join hands in meeting the common challenges.
【译文】历史表明，不同社会体制的国家能够联手迎接共同的挑战。

depress [di'pres]　　　　　　　　*vt*. 压抑；降低

【例句】What is the most serious feeling for people who are depressed?
【译文】抑郁症患者最糟糕的感觉是什么？

depressant [di'presnt]　　　　　*n*. 抑制剂
　　　　　　　　　　　a. 有镇静作用的；使消沉的

【例句】Anti-depressants work by increasing chemicals which facilitate communications between neurons in the brain.
【译文】抗抑郁药通过增加那些能促进大脑神经元之间交流的化学物质来发挥作用。

depression [di'preʃən] *n*. 不景气，萧条；沮丧，消沉

【例句】With the very extended computer use，this

isolation from the real world can lead to loneliness and even depression.

【译文】随着计算机的使用越来越广泛，这种与现实世界的隔离会导致孤独甚至抑郁。

deprive [di'praiv]　　　　　　　*vt*. 剥夺，夺去，使丧失

【搭配】be deprived of 被剥夺

【例句】And it made him determined to do something for convicts and slaves and for all who were oppressed and deprived of their liberty.

【译文】这促使他下定决心去为了罪犯和奴隶，为了所有受压迫、被剥夺了自由的人们做点儿力所能及的事。

desperate ['despərit]　　　　　　*a*. 绝望的，危急的；
　　　　　　　　　　　　　　　　不顾一切的，铤而走险的

【例句】Thousands of Mexicans arrive each day in this city, desperate for economic opportunities.

【译文】每天都有成千上万的墨西哥人到达这个城市，渴望获得发财的机会。

destination [ˌdesti'neiʃən]　　　　*n*. 目的地，终点；
　　　　　　　　　　　　　　　　　　　　目的，目标

【例句】Every year, millions of patients from around the globe flock to some of the hottest medical tourism destinations in order to receive five-star treatment.

【译文】 每年，来自世界各地的数百万患者涌向一些最热门的医疗旅游目的地，以接受五星级治疗。

detail [ˈdiːteil, diˈteil]　　　　　　*n. / vt.* 细节；说情；枝节，琐事；详述，详谈

【搭配】 in detail 详细地
【联想】 detailed *a.* 详细的

deteriorate [diˈtiəriəreit]　　　　　*v.* 恶化，变坏，蜕变

【联想】 deterioration *n.* 变坏，恶化，堕落
【例句】 Some scientists are dubious of the claim that organisms deteriorate with age as an inevitable outcome of living.
【译文】 有机组织随着年龄的增长而退化是不可避免的自然生理现象，对这一论断有科学家持怀疑态度。

detrimental [ˌdetriˈmentl]　　　　　*a.* 有害的，不利的

【例句】 The chemical was found to be detrimental to human health.
【译文】 这种化学物质被发现对人体健康有害。

diabetes [ˌdaiəˈbiːtiːz]　　　　　　　　*n.* 糖尿病

diagnose [ˈdaiəgnəuz]　　　　　　　*v.* 诊断；判断

【例句】One of my neighbors caught a bad cold and went to his doctor, who diagnosed his cold as SARS.

【译文】我的一个邻居重感冒，去看病时被医生诊断为非典型性肺炎。

diagnosis [ˌdaiəg'nəusis]　　　　*n*. 诊断；调查分析

【导学】diagnosis 复数形式为 diagnoses。

diarrhea [ˌdaiə'ri:ə]　　　　　　　　*n*. 腹泻

racial ['reiʃəl]　　　　　　*a*. 人种的，种族的

【例句】There is no racial discrimination to be felt in this city.

【译文】在这个城市里感觉不到种族歧视。

racism ['reisizəm]　*n*. 种族主义；种族歧视（意识）

radiate ['reidieit]　　　*v*.（使）闪光，发光；
　　　　　　　　　　　　　（使）辐射；（使）显出，流露

【例句】In the darkness, his eyes seemed to radiate some inner strength.

【译文】黑暗中，他的双眼似乎流露出某种内在的力量。

radical ['rædikəl]　　　　　*a*. 基本的，重要的；
　　　　　　　　　　　　　　　激进的，极端的

【例句】 Eight-year-old children have a radically different learning strategy from twelve-year-olds and adults.

【译文】 八岁孩子的学习策略与十二岁孩子和成年人截然不同。

radiologist [ˌreidiˈɔlədʒist]　　　　　*n.* 放射科医生；
　　　　　　　　　　　　　　　　　　　　　　　X光科的医生

rampant [ˈræmpənt]　　*a.* 泛滥的；猖獗的；疯长的

【例句】 Unemployment is now rampant in most of Europe.

【译文】 在欧洲的大部分地区，失业问题难以控制。

random [ˈrændəm]　　　*a.* 随机的；任意的，随便的
　　　　　　　　　　　　n. 偶然的（或随便的）行动（或过程）

【搭配】 at random 随便的，任意的

【例句】 When a psychologist does a general experiment about the human mind, he selects people at random and asks them questions.

【译文】 当心理学家做关于人类心理的普遍实验时，他通常会随机选择人来问一些问题。

range [reindʒ]　　　　　　*n.* 范围，距离，领域；
　　　　　　　　　　　　　　排列，连续，（山）脉

【搭配】 range from... to... 从……到……不等

【例句】Your Bluetooth Wireless Headset can communicate with other Bluetooth devices within a
range of approximately 10 meters (33 feet).

【译文】你的无线蓝牙耳机可在约 10 米（33 英尺）范围
内与其他蓝牙设备进行通讯。

rare [reə]　　　　　　　　 *a*. 稀有的，难得的，珍奇的；
稀薄的，稀疏的

【导学】辨析 rare, scarce：rare 指罕见的、稀奇的物
品；scarce 指寻常物的短缺。

【例句】It is a rare treasure of historical records.

【译文】这是史上罕见的史料珍品。

rarely ['reəli]　　　　　　　 *ad*. 稀少，很少，难得

【导学】rarely 放在句首时，句子需要部分倒装，和
seldom, hardly 用法相同。

【例句】Science and politics make uncomfortable bed-
fellows. Rarely is this more true than in the
case of climate change.

【译文】科学和政治是同床异梦的伙伴。很少有比气候
变化更真实的情况了。

rash [ræʃ]　　　　　　　　　 *a*. 轻率的，鲁莽的

【例句】I'm not very happy about our rash decision.

【译文】我不很赞成我们的草率决定。

rate [reit] 　　　　　*n.* 速率，比率；等级；价格，费
　　　　　　　　　　　　　　vt. 评级，评价

【搭配】at any rate 无论如何，至少

【导学】辨析 rate，ratio：rate 意为"速率，速度"，
　　　　一般用词，既可指速度又可指比率，如
　　　　survival rate（成活率）；ratio 意为"比率，
　　　　比例"，指两个同类数互相比较，其中一个数
　　　　是另一个数的几倍或几分之几，如 4 : 3。

【例句】Recycling waste slows down the rate at which we
　　　　use up the Earth's finite resources.

【译文】废物再利用减缓了我们消耗地球有限资源的速
　　　　度。

ratio [ˈreiʃiəu] 　　　　　　　　　　*n.* 比率，比

rational [ˈræʃənl] 　　　　　　　*a.* 理性的，合理的

【例句】Respecting persons，therefore，means to re-
　　　　spect them as rational creatures.

【译文】因此，尊重他人也就是尊重他们为理性人。

raw [rɔː] 　　　　*a.* 生的，未煮熟的；未加工过的

【搭配】raw material 原材料

【例句】It was reported that bacteria contaminated up
　　　　to 80% of domestic retail raw chicken in the
　　　　United States.

【译文】据报道，细菌污染了美国国内80%的零售生鸡肉。

react [ri'ækt] *vi*. 反应，起作用

【搭配】react to 对……做出反应

【例句】How do people in the UK react to the robot vacuum cleaner?

【译文】英国人对真空吸尘机器人的反响如何？

reaction [ri(ː)'ækʃən] *n*. 反应；反作用（力）

【搭配】reaction to 对……的反应

【例句】Ms. Smith's reaction to the virulent strain of E. coli was extreme.

【译文】史密斯女士对大肠杆菌的毒性菌株的反应是极端的。

readily ['redili] *ad*. 容易地；乐意地

【例句】Knowledge is more readily available on Internet-connected devices.

【译文】知识在联网设备上更容易获得。

realistic [riə'listik] *a*. 现实的，现实主义的；逼真的

【联想】unrealistic *a*. 不切实际的

【例句】Both the professional and the public should have a realistic view of what is possible.

【译文】专业人士和公众都应该对可能发生的事情有一个现实的看法。

reality [ri(ː)'æliti]　　　　　　*n*. 现实，实际；真实

【搭配】in reality 实际上，事实上

reap [riːp]　　　　　　　　　　*v*. 收割，收获

【例句】Anyone clever enough to modify this information for his own purposes can reap substantial rewards.

【译文】任何一个足够聪明的人出于个人目的修改这项资料，就能从中获取丰厚的酬劳。

rear [riə]　　　　　　　　　　*vt*. 抚养；饲养
　　　　　　　　　　n. 后部，尾部　*a*. 后方的，背后的

【搭配】at the rear of 在……的后部

【例句】The father and mother of a child did not rear their infant alone.

【译文】孩子的父亲和母亲不是独自抚养孩子的。

reasonable ['riːznəbl]　*a*. 合理的，讲理的；公道的

【例句】This statement is a reasonable conclusion looking at world politics and economics.

【译文】看看世界的政治与经济就可以说这是个合理的断言。

recall [ri'kɔːl]　　　　　　*vt*. 回想；叫回；收回

【例句】Patients can recall what they hear while under general anesthetic even if they don't wake up.

【译文】 患者即使没有醒来，也能回忆起全身麻醉时听到的声音。

---

reciprocal [ri'siprəkəl]　　　　　*a*. 相互的，互惠的

【例句】 A succession of reciprocal visits by the two countries' leaders have taken their relations out of cooler over the past 20 months.

【译文】 在过去的 20 个月里，两国领导人的一系列互访使两国关系走出了低谷。

---

recreation [rekri'eiʃ(ə)n]　　　　　*n*. 娱乐，消遣

【联想】 recreational *a*. 娱乐的

【例句】 That includes stress, diet, lifestyle choices, recreational and medicinal drug use and infections.

【译文】 那包括压力、饮食、生活方式选择、娱乐和药物使用以及感染。

---

region ['ri:dʒən]　　　　　*n*. 地区，区域；范围

【联想】 regional *a*. 区域的

【例句】 The bacteria which make the food go bad prefer to live in the watery regions of the mixture.

【译文】 能使食物变坏的细菌更喜欢在混合物的含水区域生存。

Day *10*

diet ['daiət]   *n*. 饮食，食物

【联想】dietary *a*. 饮食的

【搭配】be/go on a diet 节食

disabled [dis'eib(ə)ld]   *a*. 残疾的

【例句】Some parents learn about genetic anomalies after their disabled child is born.

【译文】一些父母在有缺陷的孩子出生后才了解到基因异常的情况。

disadvantage [ˌdisəd'vɑːntidʒ]

          n. 不利，不利条件；缺点，劣势

【例句】What is not the disadvantage of telemedicine for a doctor?

【译文】对医生来讲，哪一个不是远程医疗的缺陷？

disappointed [ˌdisə'pɔintid]   *a*. 失望的

disaster [di'zɑːstə]   *n*. 灾害，灾难，灾祸

【例句】It was called the biggest disaster in the 20th century.

【译文】这堪称 20 世纪最大的灾难。

discard [disˈkɑːd] *vt.* 丢弃，舍弃，抛弃

【例句】 Footballers are often reluctant, for superstitious reasons, to discard their old boots.

【译文】足球运动员通常因为迷信而不愿意扔掉自己的旧战靴。

discharge [disˈtʃɑːdʒ] *v. / n.* 释放；卸（货），解除，排出；允许离开；放电

【例句】 When a forest goes ablaze, it discharges hundreds of chemical compounds, including carbon monoxide.

【译文】森林起火时，会释放出数百种化合物，包括一氧化碳。

discriminate [disˈkrimineit] *vt.* (between) 区分，辨别；(against) 歧视

【导学】搭配介词：from "将……同……区分开来"，between "区分，辨别"，against "歧视，排斥"。

【例句】 However, paradoxically, just recently a group of black parents filed a lawsuit in California claiming that the state's ban on IQ testing discriminates against their children by denying them the opportunity to take the test.

【译文】 然而荒谬的是，就在最近，加州的一群黑人家长一纸诉讼，状告地方所颁布的智商测试禁令歧视黑人小孩，剥夺了孩子们参加智商测试的机会。

disseminate [di'semineit]　　　　*vt.* 散布，传播

【例句】 Publishing in scientific journals is the most common and powerful means to disseminate new research findings.

【译文】 在科学期刊上发表文章是传播新研究成果的最常见和最有力的手段。

disgrace [dis'greis]　　*n.* 耻辱，丢脸的人（或事）
　　　　　　　　　　　　　　v. 玷污

【例句】 Improved treatment has changed the outlook of HIV patients, but there is still a serious stigma (disgrace) attached to AIDS.

【译文】 治疗方案的改进改变了艾滋病人的前景，但是艾滋病仍有严重的污名。

dismay [dis'mei]　　　　*vt.* 使失望，使惊愕
　　　　　　　　　　　　　　n. 失望，气馁，惊愕

【例句】 I was dismayed at Professor Smith's comment on my paper.

【译文】 听到史密斯教授对我的论文的评价，我感到
沮丧。

dismiss [dis'mis]　　*vt.* 不再考虑；免职，解雇，
开除；解散

【例句】 As we have said on several occasions, this
option can no longer be dismissed as fantasy.

【译文】 正如我们在几次场合所说的那样，这种选择不
能再被视为幻想而不了了之了了。

dispatch/despatch [dis'pætʃ]　　*v.* 分派特定任务
n. 派遣

displace [dis'pleis]　　*vt.* 取代，替代；
迫使……离开家园，使离开原位

【例句】 Television has displaced motion picture as
America's most popular form of entertainment.

【译文】 电视取代了电影的地位，成了美国最为普遍的
娱乐方式。

distract [dis'trækt]　*vt.* 使……分心，使分散注意力

【例句】 Although we tried to concentrate on the
lecture, we were distracted by the noise from
the next room.

【译文】 尽管我们试图将注意力集中在讲座上，但隔壁

房间传来的噪声还是让我们分了神。

disturb [dis'tə:b]　　*vt.* 扰乱，妨碍；打扰，使不安

【例句】Please don't disturb me while I'm working.

【译文】请不要在我工作时打扰我。

disturbance [dis'tə:bəns]　　　　*n.* 动乱；骚扰，
干扰；（身心）失调

【例句】This disturbance would have occurred sooner or later.

【译文】这场风波迟早要来。

domain [də'mein]　　　*n.* （活动、思想等）领域，
范围；领地，势力范围

【例句】If you do not confirm this Internet domain change with your ISP, you will not be able to send or receive E-mail.

【译文】如果不与 ISP 确认该 Internet 域的更改，你将无法收发电子邮件。

dominate ['dɔmineit]　　　*vt.* 支配，统治，控制；
高出于，居高临下 *vi.* 居支配地位，处于最重要的地位

【联想】dominant *a.* 支配的，统治的，居高临下的；
显性的

【例句】In a technology-intensive enterprise, the

computer dominates all processes of production and management.

【译文】在技术密集型企业中，计算机控制着生产和管理的所有过程。

donate [dəu'neit]　　　　　　v. 捐赠，馈赠

【例句】President donated thousands of books to the local library and visited the local schools with his wife.

【译文】总统向当地的图书馆捐赠了几千本图书，并和夫人一起参观了当地的几所学校。

dramatic [drə'mætik]　　a. 引人注目的；戏剧的，戏剧性的

【例句】It turns out both are important, but the effect is most dramatic when they act together.

【译文】事实证明，两者都很重要，但当它们一起行动时，效果最为显著。

drawback ['drɔːbæk]　　n. 困难，缺点，不足之处

【例句】The same benefits and drawbacks are found when using CT scanning to detect lung cancer.

【译文】当使用 CT 扫描检测癌症时，也发现了相同的优点和缺点。

duplicate ['dju:plikeit]　　　　　　*vt*. 复制

　　　　　　　['du:plikət]　　　　　*n*. 复制品，副本

【例句】 The problem, the scientists say, is that AI has been trying to separate the highest, most abstract levels of thought, like language and mathematics, and to duplicate them with logical, step-by-step programs.

【译文】 科学家们认为，问题在于 AI 一直试图将最高级、最抽象的思维层次分离开来，如语言和数学思维，并利用逻辑程序逐步将这些思维复制。

durable ['djuərəbl]　　　　　　*a*. 耐久的

【例句】 They are often more comfortable and more durable than civilian clothes.

【译文】 它们常常比平时穿的衣服更舒适耐用。

duration [djuə'reiʃən]　　　　*n*. 持续，持续时间

eczema ['eksimə]　　　　　　　*n*. 湿疹

economical [ˌi:kə'nɔmikəl]　　*a*. 节俭的，节省的，经济的

【导学】 辨析 economic，economical：economic 表示经济的或与之有关的，经济学的或与之有关

的；economical 表示节俭的，不浪费或不挥霍的，节约的，通过高效率的运作和削减不必要的性能来节省费用的。

economy [i(:)'kɔnəmi]　　　　*n*. 经济，经济制度；节约，节省

educate ['edju(:)keit]　　　　*vt*. 教育，培养，训练

【例句】An educator must first educate himself.

【译文】教育者必须自己先受教育。

effective [i'fektiv]　　　　*a*. 有效的，生效的

【导学】辨析 effective，efficient，valid：effective 表示有效的，具有预期或先见效果的，既强调产生满意的效果，又注重不浪费时间、精力等因素，因此往往带有"有效率的"意味；efficient 意为"有能力的；高效率的"；valid 表示（法律上）有效的，正当的，或在一段时间、某种情况下有效的。

【例句】A proven method for effective textbook reading is the SQ3R method.

【译文】经过证明的一种有效的阅读课本的方法是 SQ3R 方法。

elaborate [i'læbərət]　　　　　　*a.* 精细的，详尽的
　　　　　　　[i'læbəreit]　　　　　　*v.* 详细描述

【例句】They had created elaborate computer programs to run the system.

【译文】他们创造了非常精细的计算机程序来运行这个系统。

elastic [i'læstik]　　　　　　*n.* 橡皮圈，松紧带
　　　　a. 有弹性的，弹力的；灵活的，可伸缩的

【例句】Our plans are still very elastic.

【译文】我们的计划仍然是有弹性的。

elevate ['eliveit] *vt.* 提升……的职位，提高，改善；
　　　　　　使情绪高昂，使兴高采烈；举起，使上升

【导学】近义词：hoist，heave，tilt，levitate，raise；
　　　　advance，upgrade，further，promote

【例句】Second，will male-dominated companies elevate women to higher-paid jobs as they elevate men?

【译文】其二，男性一统天下的公司会像他们提拔男性一样提拔女性到高薪岗位吗？

eliminate [i'limineit]　　　　*vt.* 消灭，除去，排出

【例句】She has been eliminated from the swimming

race because she did not win any of the practice races.

【译文】她已被取消了参加游泳比赛的资格，因为她在训练中没有得到名次。

embrace [im'breis]　　　*vt.* 抱，拥抱；包括，包含；包围，环绕

【例句】Expanding cities must embrace such technologies and strategies.

【译文】城市的扩张必须采用这样的技术和策略。

emigrate ['emigreit]　　　*vi.* 移居外国，移民

emit [i'mit] *vt.* 发出，发射；散发（光、热、气味等）

【联想】emission *n.* 排放，散发

【例句】The report is expected to start labeling phones with data on the amount of radiation they emit.

【译文】该报告预计将开始为手机贴上辐射量数据标签。

emotion [i'məuʃən]　　　*n.* 情感，情绪

【导学】emotion, feeling, passion：emotion 一般指比较强烈、深刻且能感动人的感情或情绪，多含精神上的反应，如爱、惧、哀、乐等；feeling 泛指人体的一切感觉、情绪和心情；

passion 意为"激情",指往往由于正确的判断受其影响而表现出强烈的或激烈的情绪,有时不能自持,甚至失去理智。

【例句】Love,hatred,and grief are emotions.

【译文】爱、恨、悲伤都是感情。

emphasis ['emfəsis]　　　　　　　*n*. 强调,重点

【搭配】lay/put/place emphasis on/upon 注重,着重于,强调

【导学】 emphasis 复数形式为 emphases(参见 analysis)。

emphasize ['emfəsaiz]　　　　　*vt*. 强调,着重

【例句】Advertisements showed pictures of the beautiful scenery that could be enjoyed along some of the more famous western routes and emphasized the romantic names of some of these trains(Empire Builder,etc).

【译文】广告展示了在沿途能够欣赏的一些有名的西部线路美丽景色的图片,而且还重点强调了一些火车的名字(帝国建造者等)。

enable [i'neibl]　　　　　　　*vt*. 使能够,使可能

【搭配】enable sb. to do 使某人能做

endeavour [in'devə]　　　*vi*. 努力，尽力，尝试

【导学】近义词：attempt，aim，essay，strive，try，effort

【例句】Apart from philosophical and legal reasons for respecting patients' wishes, there are several practical reasons why doctors should endeavor to involve patients in their own medical care decisions.

【译文】除了在道义上和法律方面要求尊重患者的愿望之外，之所以医生努力让患者参与自己的医疗护理决策，还有不少现实的原因。

engage [in'geidʒ]　　　*vt*. 使从事，使忙于；占用（时间等）；雇用，聘用；使订婚　*vi*. 从事于，参加

【搭配】be engaged in 正忙于，从事于

　　　　be engaged to 与……订婚

enhance [in'hɑːns]　　　*vt*. 提高；增强

【例句】The existing HIV drugs will be enhanced to be more effective in 25 years.

【译文】25年后，现存的艾滋病药物会得以改良，药效更好。

regulate ['regjuleit]　　　*vt*. 管理，控制；调整，调节，校准

【例句】 The speed of the machine may be automatically regulated to pace the packing operation by an inner microcomputer.

【译文】 机器的速度可通过内部的微型电脑自动调节得同包装速度一致。

regulation [regju'leiʃən]　*n*. 管理，控制；规章，规则

【搭配】 adopt new regulations 采取新规定
break/violate a regulation 违反规定
obey/observe regulations 遵守规定

relate [ri'leit]　　　*vi*. 联系，关联 *vt*. 叙述，讲述

【搭配】 be related to 与……有关

【例句】 These things often are stress-related, but we're still going to do a few blood tests just to rule a few things out.

【译文】 这些事情通常与压力有关，但我们仍要做一些血液测试，以排除一些可能。

related [ri'leitid]　　　*a*. 叙述的，讲述的；有关系的

relationship [ri'leiʃənʃip]　　　*n*. 关系，联系

【联想】 relation *n*. 关系

relax [ri'læks]　　　*vt*. 使放松，使休息；缓和，放宽
vi. 放松，休息；松弛

release [ri'li:s]　　　　　　　　　*vt*. 释放，放出；发布，
　　　　　　　　　　　　　　　发行；放开，松开

【例句】 Websites are established for students to release their depression and report anonymously their own problems.

【译文】 网站建设的目的是为了让学生释放压抑的情绪，还可以匿名报告自己的问题。

relevant ['relivənt]　　　　　　　*a*. (to) 相关的，切题的；
　　　　　　　　　　　　　　　适当的，中肯的

【例句】 This could be relevant as ulcers may run in the family.

【译文】 这可能有关系，因为溃疡是可以在家族中遗传的。

reliable [ri'laiəbl]　　　　　　　　　　*a*. 可靠的

reluctant [ri'lʌktənt]　　　　　　　*a*. 不情愿的，勉强的

【联想】 reluctance *n*. 不情愿（近义词：unwillingness）

【例句】 He wanted to stay at home, but at last he agreed, very reluctantly though, to go to the concert.

【译文】 他想待在家里，但是最后还是非常勉强地同意出席音乐会。

【例句】Sometimes we gaze through a subject and are reluctant to stop for too much detail.

【译文】有时我们凝视物品，不愿意为太多的细节而驻足。

rely [ri'lai]   *vi*. 依靠，信赖，依仗

【搭配】rely on/upon 依靠；信赖

【例句】The poor used to rely on government aid.

【译文】穷人过去都依靠政府的救助。

remark [ri'mɑːk]   *n*. 评语，意见 *vt*. 说，评论
vi. 议论，评论

【搭配】remark on/upon 就某事发表意见

remarkable [ri'mɑːkəbl]   *a*. 值得注意的；
显著的，异常的，非凡的

【例句】A newspaper is even more remarkable for the way one reads it.

【译文】报纸对于读者来说，阅读的方式是更值得注意的。

repetition [ˌrepi'tiʃən]   *n*. 重复，反复；背诵

【联想】repeatedly *ad*. 重复地

【例句】If the work of remedying of any defect or damage may affect the performance of the works, the engineer may require the repetition of any of the tests described in the contract.

【译文】如果任何缺陷或损害的修补工作可能影响到工程运行时，工程师可要求重新进行合同中列明的任何测试。

replace [ri(ː)'pleis] *vt.* 放回；替换，取代

【联想】replacement *n.* 取代，替换

【搭配】replace... with... 以……代替……

【导学】辨析 replace，substitute：replace 指取代、替换陈旧的、用坏的或遗失的东西，用法是 replace A with B（用 B 代替 A）；substitute 指用一件东西替换另一件东西，用法是 substitute B for A（用 B 代替 A）。

【例句】The new city, Brasilia, replaced Rio de Janeiro as the capital of Brazil in 1960.

【译文】1960 年，巴西利亚这座新城市取代了里约热内卢成为巴西的首都。

repopulate [ˌriː'pɔːpjuleit] *vt.* 重新入住，再生

represent [ˌriːpri'zent] *vt.* 表示，阐明，说明；描写，表现，象征；代理，代表

【搭配】represent... as 把……描述成

【例句】They elected him to represent them.

【译文】他们选他当代表。

representative [repri'zentətiv]

　　　　　　　　　　　　a. 典型的，有代表性的

　　　　　　　　　　　　n. 代表，代理人

【搭配】be representative of 有代表性的，典型的

reputation [repju'teiʃn]　　　　　　*n.* 名声，声望

【搭配】have a reputation for 因……而出名

　　　　gain/acquire/establish a reputation 博得名声

reserve [ri'zə:v]　　　　　　　*vt.* 储备；保留；预订

　　n. 储备品，储备金，储备；保留地；节制，谨慎

【联想】reservation *n.* 预订，保留

【搭配】without reserve 毫无保留地

【例句】I reserved a tennis court, but it's taken over by someone else.

【译文】我预订了一个网球场，但被别人占了。

Day *11*

entertain [ˌentəˈtein] *vt.* 使欢乐，使娱乐；招待，款待

【联想】 entertainment *n.* 娱乐，文娱节目，表演会；
招待，款待，请客

enthusiasm [inˈθjuːziæzəm] *n.* 热情，热心，积极性

【联想】 enthusiastic *a.* 热情的

【例句】 From a broad education to interdisciplinary
study, we can see the enthusiasm for breadth
of knowledge.

【译文】 从通识教育到跨学科研究，我们可以看到对知
识广度的热情。

environment [inˈvaiərənmənt] *n.* 环境，四周，外界

【联想】 environmental *a.* 环境的

【例句】 Radical environmentalists have blamed pollu-
tants and synthetic chemicals in pesticides for
the disruption of human hormones.

【译文】 激进的环保主义者指责杀虫剂中的污染物和合
成化学物质破坏了人类荷尔蒙。

equivalent [iˈkwivələnt] *a.* 相等的；等价的，等量的
n. 同等物，等价物，对等

【例句】A mile is equivalent to about 1. 6 kilometers.

【译文】1 英里大约等于1.6 千米。

eradicate [i'rædikeit]   *v*. 根除

【导学】近义词：extirpate, exterminate, annihilate;
abolish, destroy

establish [is'tæbliʃ]   *n*. 建立，设立，创办;
确立，使确认

【联想】establishment *n*. 建立，设立，确立；建立的
机构（组织）

【例句】The Minister established a commission to suggest improvements in the educational system.

【译文】部长组织了一个研究组，为改进教育制度提供
建议。

estimate ['estimeit]   *vt*. 估计，估价，评价
['estimət]   *n*. 估计，估价，评价

【联想】estimation *n*. 估计，预估

【例句】The overall fat content can then be estimated
from the body's resistance.

【译文】然后就可以根据身体的抵抗力来估计脂肪总量。

essence ['esns]   *n*. 本质，实质；精华，精粹

【例句】For most thinkers since the Greek philoso-
phers, it was self-evident that there is some-

131

thing called human nature, something that constitutes the essence of man.

【译文】不言而喻，对于希腊哲学家及其后的大多数思想家来说，有一种叫作人性的东西，构成了人的本质。

ethical ['eθikl]　　　　　*a*.（有关）道德的；伦理的；合乎道德的

【联想】unethical *a*. 不道德的

【例句】Leading an ethical, principled life was important.

【译文】过一种有道德、有原则的生活很重要。

evaluate [i'væljueit]　　　　　*vt*. 评价，评估

【例句】The proposal could not be evaluated because the details had not been published.

【译文】还不能评估这个建议，因为细节还没有披露。

evolve [i'vɔlv]　　　　*v*.（使）进化，（使）演化；（使）发展，（使）演变

【联想】evolution *n*. 进化，演化；发展，渐进

【例句】The developmental history of the society tells us that man has evolved from the ape.

【译文】社会发展史告诉我们：人是从类人猿进化来的。

exaggerate [ig'zædʒəreit]   *v.* 夸张，夸大

【例句】 They exaggerated the function of the medicine.
【译文】 他们夸大了这个药品的功能。

exchange [iks'tʃeindʒ] *vt.* 交换，交流；调换，兑换
                                              n. 交换台，交易所

【搭配】 exchange A for B/substitute A for B
        用 A 去换 B

excitement [ik'saitmənt]   *n.* 刺激，兴奋

【联想】 excite *v.* 激动；exciting *a.* 令人激动的；
        excited *v.* 感到激动的
【例句】 She, a crazy fan, felt a tingle of excitement
        at the sight of Michael Jackson.
【译文】 她是个狂热的粉丝，看到迈克尔·杰克逊时感
        到一阵狂喜。

exhaust [ig'zɔːst]   *vt.* 用尽，耗尽，竭力；
                    使衰竭，使精疲力竭 *n.* 排气装置；废气

【联想】 exhausting *a.* 令人精疲力竭的；exhausted *a.*
        感到精疲力竭的；exhaustive *a.* 详尽的
【例句】 Exhaustion syndrome is the typical represent-
        ative of being subhealthy.
【译文】 "疲劳综合征"就是亚健康状态的典型代表。

expand [iks'pænd]　　　　　*vt.* 使膨胀，详述，扩张
　　　　　　　　　　　　　　　　vi. 张开，发展

【例句】Dance training improves thinking though mimicry and acting classes seem to expand language.

【译文】舞蹈训练会改进思维，而模仿和表演课会扩展语言。

expansion [iks'pænʃən]　　　　*n.* 扩充，开展，膨胀

experimental [iksˌperi'mentl]　　　*a.* 试验（上）的

【联想】experiment *n.* 试验

【例句】However，they are very much in the experimental stage.

【译文】然而，他们仍处于试验阶段。

explode [iks'pləud]　　*v.* （使）爆炸，爆发，破裂

【搭配】explode with anger 勃然大怒，大发脾气
　　　　explode with laughter 哄堂大笑

【例句】It was during the morning rush hour that the bomb exploded.

【译文】爆炸是在早高峰时发生的。

exploit [iks'plɔit]　　*vt.* 使用，利用；开采，开发

【例句】Many Countries exploit oil under the sea.

【译文】许多国家在海底开采石油。

explore [iks'plɔ:]　　　*vt.* 探险；探索，探究；勘探

【例句】Play is the most powerful way a child explores the world and learns about himself.

【译文】玩耍是孩子探索世界和了解自身的最有力的方法。

external [iks'tə:nl]　　　　　　*a.* 外部的，外面的

【例句】They also need significant increases in external financing and technical support.

【译文】他们还需要大幅度增加外部资助和技术支持。

extraordinary [iks'trɔ:dnri]　　*a.* 非常的，特别的

extract [iks'trækt]　　*vt.* 取出，抽出，拔出；提取，提炼，榨取；获得，索取；摘录，抄录
　　　　　['ekstrækt]　*n.* 摘录，选段；提出物，精华，汁

【例句】It is one thing to locate oil，but it is quite another to extract and transport it to the industrial centers.

【译文】找到石油是一回事，提炼并把石油运送到工业中心却完全是另一回事。

facilitate [fə'siliteit]　　　　*vt.* 使便利；促进，帮助

【例句】 The automatic doors in supermarkets facilitate the entry and exit of customers with
shopping carts.

【译文】 超市的自动门给推购物车出入的顾客提供了
便利。

facility [fə'siliti]　　　　*n.* 便利；(*pl.*) 设备，设施

【导学】 作"设施"讲时，要用复数形式。

【例句】 In the meeting, the government officer promised
an improvement in hospitals and other health
care facilities.

【译文】 在会上，政府官员许诺对医院和其他医疗健康
设施进行改善。

factor ['fæktə]　　　　　　　　　　*n.* 因素，要素

【例句】 The risk factors for long-term criminality can
be spotted in kindergarten.

【译文】 未来犯罪的危险因素在幼儿园阶段就可以发现。

faculty ['fækəlti]　　　　*n.* 才能，本领，能力；
　　　　　　　　　　　　　　　全体教师；院，系

【搭配】 have a faculty for sth. 有做某事的才能

【导学】 做主语时，看作整体，谓语用单数形式；看
作个体，谓语用复数形式。

【例句】 The average number of the faculty of law in every city is forty-five.

【译文】 在每个城市中平均有 45 所法学院。

fade [feid]   *vi*. 褪色；逐渐消失

【例句】 The ability is also one of the first visual aptitudes to fade with age.

【译文】 这个能力也是最早随着年龄增长而减退的视觉能力之一。

failure ['feiljə]   *n*. 失败，不及格；失败者；没做到；失灵

【联想】 fail *v*. 失败；fail to do 未能做成某事

【例句】 I believe that only such efforts can save us from the social trends, political movements, and policy failures that are elevating our risk of a pandemic.

【译文】 我认为，只有这样的努力才能使我们免受社会趋势、政治运动和政策失败的影响，而这些都会提高我们经历大流行病的风险。

fame [feim]   *n*. 名声，名望

【例句】 Her story shows an indifference to honors and fame can lead to great achievements.

【译文】 她的故事表明，不计较荣誉和名声也能够取得巨大的成就。

fancy ['fænsi] *n.* 想象 (力); 爱好, 迷恋 *a.* 别致的; 异想天开的 *v.* 想象, 幻想; 想要, 喜欢; 相信; 猜想

【搭配】 take a fancy to 爱好, 爱上
have a fancy for 热衷于

【导学】 后接动名词, 不接动词不定式 fancy doing。

fantastic [fæn'tæstik] *a.* 空想的; 奇异的, 古怪的

【联想】 fantasy *n.* 异想天开

【例句】 It is simply a fantastic imagination to master a foreign language overnight.

【译文】 想在一夜之间掌握一门外语真是异想天开。

fare [fɛə] *n.* 车费, 船费

【导学】 辨析 fare, fee, charge: fare 指交通费用; fee 指一种法律或组织机构规定的为某项特权而征收的固定费用, 如会费、学费、入场费、报名费、手续费等, 也指对职业性的服务所支付的报酬, 如医生的诊费、代理人佣金、律师的胜诉金等; charge 指购买货物所付出的价钱, 或获得服务所付出的费用。

fascinating ['fæsineitiŋ] *a.* 迷人的, 醉人的

fatal ['feitl] *n.* 致命的, 毁灭性的

【联想】 fatality *n.* 致命性

【例句】 About 90,000 people were infected — hundreds
fatally — in five countries.

【译文】 五个国家中大约9万人感染，数百人有致命危险。

fate [feit]   *n*. 命运

【导学】 辨析 fate, destiny：fate 指不可避免的命运，
尤指不幸的命运；destiny 指预先注定的命
运，宿命。

fatigue [fə'ti:g]   *n*. 疲乏，劳累

【例句】 This pill will work wonders for fatigue.

【译文】 这种药片对（缓解）疲劳有神奇的效果。

faulty ['fɔːlti]   *a*. 有错误的，有缺点的

【例句】 Their arguments were based on faulty reasoning.

【译文】 他们的论点基于错误的推理。

favo(u)rable ['feivərəbl]

                    a. 顺利的，有利的；称赞的，赞成的

【搭配】 be favorable for 对某事有利

be favorable to 赞同；（对某人）有利，有益

【例句】 This is the favorable weather for working outside.

【译文】 这是适合户外工作的天气。

favo(u)rite ['feivərit]   *a*. 最喜爱的
                    n. 最喜爱的人或物

【例句】 Fishing is his favorite pastime on a hot summer day.

【译文】 在炎热的夏日，他最喜欢的休闲方式是钓鱼。

fearful ['fiəful]　*a.* 吓人的，可怕的；害怕的，担心的

feasible ['fi:zəbl]　　　　　*a.* 可行的，可能的

【例句】 His surgical procedure should succeed, for it seems quite feasible.

【译文】 他的手术应该能成功，因为听上去很可行。

feature ['fi:tʃə]　*n.* 特征，特色；面貌，容貌；特写

【例句】 Genetic features decide what you should eat for the sake of health.

【译文】 你的基因特征决定了你吃什么才能健康。

federal ['fedərəl]　　　　*a.* 联邦的，联盟的，联合的

fee [fi:]　　　　　　　　*n.* 酬金；手续费；学费

feedback ['fi:dbæk]　　　　　　　*n.* 反馈

【例句】 Eight-year-olds learn primarily from positive feedback, whereas negative feedback scarcely causes any alarm bell to ring.

【译文】 8岁的孩子主要从正面反馈中学习，而负面反馈几乎不会敲响任何警钟。

female [ˈfiːmeil] 　　　　　　　　*n.* 女子，雌性动物
　　　　　　　　　　　　　　　　　a. 女性的，雌性的

fertile [ˈfəːtail] 　　　　　　　*a.* 肥沃的，富饶的；
　　　　　　　　　　　　　　　　　　多产的，丰富的

【例句】All the flowers are grown in the fertile soil.

【译文】所有的花都生长在肥沃的土壤里。

fertilizer [ˌfəːtiˈlaizə] 　　　　*n.* 化肥，肥料

finance [faiˈnæns] 　　　　　　*n.* 财政，金融
　　　　　　　　　　　　　　　　　vt. 提供资金，接济

【联想】financial *a.* 财政的，金融的

【例句】One U.S. dollar is comparable to 131 Japanese yen according to *China Daily*'s finance news report yesterday.

【译文】据昨天《中国日报》财经新闻报道，1 美元可兑换 131 日元。

resist [riˈzist] 　　　　*vt.* 抵抗，反抗；忍住，抵制

【联想】resistance *n.* 抵抗，反抗

【例句】We must raise the capacity to resist corruption.

【译文】我们必须提高反腐能力。

resistant [riˈzistənt] 　　　　　*a.* 抵抗的，反抗的

【搭配】be resistant to 对……有抵抗力的

【例句】The researchers are already working with food companies，keen to see if their products can be made resistant to bacterial attack through alterations to the food's structure.

【译文】研究人员已经和食品公司联合起来，希望他们的产品能通过改变食品的结构来抵抗细菌的侵袭。

retail ['ri:teil]　　　　　　 *n.* 零售 *a.* 零售的 *v.* 零售

【搭配】sell by/at retail 零售

retain [ri'tein]　　　　　　　　　　 *vt.* 保持，保留

【例句】People can retain conscious or subconscious memories of thoughts that happened while they were being operated on.

【译文】人们对自己手术期间发生的事情保留有意识或潜意识记忆。

retreat [ri'tri:t]　　　　　　　　　　 *vi.* 撤退，退却

【例句】Is the profession of medicine in retreat?

【译文】医学专业在衰退吗？

retrieve [ri'tri:v]　　　　 *vt.* 重新得到，取回；挽回，补救；检索

【例句】The dog was intelligent and quickly learned to retrieve the game killed by the hunter.

【译文】那狗很聪明，很快就学会了找回猎人杀死的

猎物。

reveal [ri'viːl] *vt*. 揭示，揭露，展现；告诉，泄露

【例句】 Our investigation also reveals that many companies choose not to disclose data.

【译文】 我们的研究还显示，很多公司选择不披露数据。

revelation [ˌrevi'leiʃən] *n*. 揭示，透露，启示；被揭示的真相，新发现

【例句】 "Spilling the beans" means confessing or making a startling revelation.

【译文】 "撒了豆子"意思是坦白交代或者透露惊人的真相。

reverse [ri'vəːs] *v*. 颠倒，翻转，后退
n./*a*. 反面（的），颠倒（的），相反（的）

【例句】 The technical fix does help reverse the obesity epidemic.

【译文】 科技手段确实有助于扭转肥胖流行。

rival ['raivəl] *vt*. 竞争，与……抗衡
a. 竞争的 *n*. 竞争对手

【例句】 Of all the flowers in the garden few can rival the lily.

【译文】 在花园的所有花卉中，很少有花能与百合花媲美。

romantic [rəu'mæntik]   *a*. 浪漫的，传奇的；
不切实际的，好幻想的

rural ['ruər(ə)l]   *a*. 农村的

【例句】More people live in cities than in rural areas.
The current rate of urbanization is
unprecedented in our history.

【译文】居住在城市的人多于农村，目前的城镇化速度
在我们的历史上前所未有。

Day *12*

flaw [flɔː] 　　　　　　　　　　*n*. 缺点，裂纹，瑕疵

【例句】 The statue would be perfect but for a few small flaws in its base.

【译文】 要不是基底部分有一些小的瑕疵，这座雕塑就很完美了。

【导学】 近义词：defect，imperfection，blemish，stain

forbid [fəˈbid] 　　　　　　　　*vt*. 禁止，不许，不准

【搭配】 forbid sb. to do sth. 禁止某人做某事

【联想】 prohibit sb. from doing sth., prevent sb. from doing sth., stop sb. from doing sth. 禁止某人做某事

【例句】 Waterway traffic is forbidden except on weekends.

【译文】 除了周末，水上交通工具都是禁行的。

forecast [ˈfɔːkɑːst] 　　　　　　*vt*. / *n*. 预测，预报

【导学】 辨析 forecast，predict，foretell：forecast 强调"预报"，指通过分析一些相关的信息、数据来预测，这种预测是建立在科学知识或判断上的；predict 常指根据已知的事实或自然

规律推断出未来的事情，可用于各种不同的场合；foretell 指凭借自己的经验或猜测能实现感觉到将来会发生的事情。

formal [ˈfɔːməl]　　a. 正式的；礼仪上的；形式的

【联想】informal a. 不正式的

【例句】Physician specialty is a measure of formal training in the field.

【译文】医师的专业度是该领域正式培训的一种衡量标准。

formation [fɔːˈmeiʃən] n. 构成；组织，形成物；地岩层

former [ˈfɔːmə]　　a. 在前的，以前的 n. 前者

【搭配】the former...the latter 前者……后者

formula [ˈfɔːmjulə]　　　n. 公式，程式

【搭配】formula for... ……的配方

【导学】formula 复数形式有：formulas，formulae。

formulate [ˈfɔːmjuleit]　　　　　vt. 制定；明确地表达；简洁陈述，阐明

【例句】Climate scientists will agree，their role is not to formulate policy.

【译文】气候科学家会同意，他们的角色不是制定政策。

fortunately [ˈfɔːtʃənətli]　　　　　ad. 幸亏

foundation [faun'deiʃən]　　　*n.* 成立，建立，创办；
基础，地基；根据；基金会

【搭配】lay a solid foundation for 为……打下坚实的
基础

【例句】The television station is supported by dona-
tion from foundations and other sources.

【译文】电视台接受来自各种基金会和其他来源的捐款
的支持。

fraction ['frækʃən] *n.* 碎片，小部分，一点儿；分数

【导学】辨析 fraction，part，portion，section，
segment，share：fraction 意为"小部分，
碎片"，常表示可以略去不计的微小部分；
part 纯粹为部分，并无比例内涵；portion
意为"一部分，一份"，指在某物中所占的
份额、比例；section 指通过或似乎通过切
割或分离而形成的部分，如书、文章或城市
的某一部分；segment 可与 section 换用，但
更强调某物以自然的分裂线分开的部分，或
因其结构性质而分裂的部分；share 指所分
享、分担的一部分，强调共性。

【例句】You could try medical tourism and receive
quality care for a fraction of the price and
without the long wait.

【译文】你可以尝试医疗旅游，只需花费一小部分的价

格就可以得到优质的护理，而无须漫长的等待。

fracture ['fræktʃə]　　　　　　*n.* 破裂，骨折
　　　　　　　　　　　　　　　v. (使) 破碎，(使) 破裂

【例句】 There is a hemi-fracture. It's not very serious, but you should take a month off work and rest in bed.

【译文】 这里有一处半骨折。虽然不严重，但你应该休假一个月，卧床休息。

fragile ['frædʒail]　　　　*a.* 脆的；虚弱的；易碎的

【例句】 Dispossessed peasants slash and burn their way into the rain forests of Latin America, and hungry nomads turn their herds out onto fragile African grassland, reducing it to desert.

【译文】 被剥夺得一无所有的农民在拉丁美洲的热带雨林中砍伐和焚烧，而饥饿的游牧民族把他们的家畜赶进了脆弱的非洲草原，使其退化成沙漠。

fragment ['frægmənt]　　　　*n.* 碎片，小部分，片断

【例句】 When she heard the news, she dropped the bowl on the floor and it broke into fragments.

【译文】 听到这个消息时，她手里的碗掉落在地，摔成碎片。

frustrate [frʌs'treit] *vt.* 破坏，阻挠；使失败，使泄气

【例句】After three hours' frustrating delay, the train at last arrived.

【译文】经过 3 个小时令人心烦的耽搁后，火车终于到达了目的地。

fundamental [ˌfʌndə'mentl] *a.* 基础的，根本的，重要的 *n.* (*pl.*) 基本原则，基本原理

【搭配】be fundamental to 对……必不可少

【联想】be essential to, be vital to 对……至关重要

【例句】These experts say that we must understand the fundamental relation between ourselves and wild animals.

【译文】这些专家说，我们必须明白我们自己和野生动物之间的重要关系。

fungal ['fʌŋgl] *a.* 真菌的；真菌引起的

【例句】Professional footballers seem as likely to suffer from fungal infections of the foot as other people.

【译文】职业足球运动员似乎和其他人一样容易患足部真菌感染。

gap [gæp] *n.* 缺口，间隔；隔阂，差距

【搭配】bridge the gap between 弥合（……之间的）

差别；消除隔阂；bridge/fill/stop/close a gap 弥补不足；填补空白

【例句】There are wide gaps in my knowledge of history.

【译文】我很缺乏历史知识。

gas [gæs]　　　　　　　　　*n.* 煤气；气体；汽油

【联想】gasoline *n.* 汽油

gastric ['gæstrik]　　　　　　　*a.* 胃的；胃部的

gear [giə]　　　　*n.* 齿轮，传动装置；用具，装备
　　　　　　　　　　　　　　　　v. 开动，连接

【搭配】gear up（使）准备好，（使）做好安排
　　　　gear... to 使……适合

【例句】Education should be geared to children's needs.

【译文】教育应适合孩子们的需要。

gene [dʒi:n]　　　　　　　　　　　*n.* 基因

【例句】Most of us inherit half our gene from our mothers and half from our fathers.

【译文】我们大多数人继承一半母亲的基因，一半父亲的基因。

generalize ['dʒenərəlaiz]　　*v.* 概括，归纳，推断

【联想】generalized 是形容词，意为"广泛的，普及的"。

【例句】 In the emic approach the researchers might choose to focus only on middle-class white families without regard for whether the information obtained in the study can be generalized or is appropriate for ethnic minority groups.

【译文】 使用主位法，研究者可能只注意到那些白人中产阶级家庭，全然不考虑研究中所获得信息是否有普遍性或者对少数民族群体是否合适。

genetic [dʒi'netik]   *a*. 遗传的，起源的

【例句】 The human population contains a great variety of genetic variation, but drugs are tested on just a few thousand people.

【译文】 人类具有各种各样的遗传变异，可是药品的试验只能在数千人中进行。

generally ['dʒenərəli]   *ad*. 一般，通常

generate ['dʒenəreit]   *vt*. 产生，发生；引起，导致

【例句】 When coal burns, it generates heat.

【译文】 煤燃烧时，产生热量。

generator ['dʒenəreitə]   *n*. 发电机，发生器

generous ['dʒenərəs]   *a*. 慷慨的，大方的；丰盛的，丰富的；宽厚的

【搭配】 be generous to sb. 对某人宽大；be generous with sth. 用某物大方

【例句】 He made such a generous contribution to the university that they are naming one of the new buildings after him.

【译文】 他给大学如此慷慨的捐助，所以他们将以他的名字给其中一座新楼命名。

---

genius [ˈdʒiːnjəs]   *n.* 天才

【联想】 have a faculty for，have a gift for，have a talent for，have a capacity for 具有……的才能/天赋

【导学】 辨析 genius，gift，talent：genius 指天赋，超常的智力和创造力，具有这种天赋的人极为罕见；gift 指天资，才能，通常被认为是生来就有的某一方面突出的才能；talent 指生来即有的天分或能力，通常需要加以培养和发展。

【例句】 I was going to be a complete engineer, technical genius and sensitive humanist all in one.

【译文】 我想做一个真正意义上的工程师，技术上的天才和敏感的人文学者集于一身的工程师。

---

genuine [ˈdʒenjuin]   *a.* 真实的，真正的；真心的，真诚的

【例句】 The questions usually grow out of their genuine interest or curiosity.

【译文】 问题通常来自他们真正的兴趣或好奇心。

global ['gləubəl]　　　　　*a*. 地球的，全球的；全局的

globe [gləub]　　　　　*n*. 地球；地球仪，球体

【例句】 We believe it is a reasonable real-world test of good manners around the globe.

【译文】 我们相信这是一个世界范围内的、合理的、现实的关于礼貌的测试。

gradual ['grædjuəl]　　　　　*a*. 逐渐的，逐步的

graduate ['grædjuət]　　　　　*n*. 毕业生；研究生
　　　　　　　['grædʒueit]　　　　　*vi*. 毕业

【联想】 undergraduate *n*. 大学本科生；postgraduate *n*. 研究生；bachelor *n*. 学士；master *n*. 硕士；doctor，Ph. D *n*. 博士

【例句】 23-year-old Eric graduated from college last year.

【译文】 23 岁的埃里克去年从大学毕业了。

grant [grɑ:nt]　*n*. 拨款；准许 *v*. 准予，授予，同意

【搭配】 take...for granted 认为……理所当然

【例句】The government gave us a grant to build another classroom.

【译文】政府给了我们一笔补助，用来盖另外一间教室。

guarantee [ˌɡærən'tiː]　　　　　*n.* 保证，保证书
　　　　　　　　　　　　　　　　　vt. 保证，担保

【导学】辨析 guarantee，pledge，warranty：guarantee 意为"担保，保证，抵押品"，指对事物的品质或人的行为提出担保，常暗示双方有法律上或其他方式的默契，保证补偿不履行所造成的损失；pledge 意为"保证，誓约，抵押品"，为普通用语，可泛指保证忠实于某种原则或接受并尽忠某一职责的庄严保证或诺言，但这都是以跟人的信誉作保证的承诺；warranty 指"（商品的）保证书，保单，保证"，如修理或退换残缺货物等。

【例句】Nuclear power，with all its inherent problems，is still the only option to guarantee enough energy in the future.

【译文】虽然核动力还存在它固有的问题，但它仍然是将来有足够能源的唯一保证。

guidance [ˈɡaidəns]　　　　　　　*n.* 引导，指导

【搭配】under the guidance of 在……引导之下

【例句】Parental guidance is crucial to the development of healthy sleep habits in children.

【译文】父母的指导对儿童养成健康的睡眠习惯至关重要。

pace [peis]　　　　　　　*n.* (一) 步，步子；步速，速度

【搭配】keep/lead pace with (与……) 并驾齐驱，保持一致；set the pace 起带头作用

【导学】辨析 pace，rate，speed，velocity：pace 意为"步速，速度，进度"，也指运动的速率，多指走路的人、跑步的人或小跑的马匹的行速，用于比喻时指各种活动、生产效率等发展的速度；rate 意为"速率，比率"，用与其他事物的关系来衡量速度、价值、成本等，作速度讲时强调单位时间内的速度；speed 意为"速率，速度"，指任何事物持续运动时的速度，尤指车辆等无生命事物的运动速度；velocity 意为"速度"，技术用语，指物体沿着特定方向运动时的速率。

【例句】Some critics question whether the quality of service has kept pace with the rapid expansion of telemedicine.

【译文】一些批评人士质疑服务质量是否跟得上远程医疗的快速扩张。

package [ˈpækidʒ]　　　　　　*n.* 包装，包裹，箱；
　　　　　　　　　　　　　　　　一揽子交易（或计划、建议等）

【搭配】a package deal/offer 一揽子交易

pact [pækt]　　　　　　　　　　*n.* 协定，条约；契约

【例句】The trade pact between those two countries come to an end.

【译文】那两个国家的通商协定宣告结束。

painful [ˈpeinfl]　　　　　　　　*a.* 痛苦的，疼痛的；
　　　　　　　　　　　　　　　　困难，令人不快的

【例句】The most painful for a lot of people is the feeling that you are useless.

【译文】对许多人来说，最痛苦的事莫过于你觉得自己无用。

palm [pɑːm]　　　　　　　　　　　*n.* 手掌

【搭配】palm off 用欺骗手段把……卖掉；grease/oil one's palm 贿赂某人；have an itching palm 贪财；in the palm of one's hand 在某人的完全控制之下；know sth. like the palm of one's hand 对某事了如指掌

pandemic [pænˈdemik]　　　　*n.* （全国或全球性）
　　　　　　　　　　　　　　　　流行病；大流行病
　　　　a.（疾病）大流行的；普遍的，全世界的

【例句】Experts say that global cooperation is essential for pandemic control.

【译文】专家表示，全球合作对疫情控制至关重要。

panel ['pænl] *n.* 专门小组；面板，控制板，仪表盘

panic ['pænik] *n.* 惊慌，恐慌 *a.* 恐慌的，惊慌的

paradox ['pærədɔks] *n.* 似乎矛盾而（可能）正确的说法；自相矛盾的人（或事情）

【例句】We work to make money, but it's a paradox that people who work hard and long often don't make the most money.

【译文】我们工作是为了挣钱，但矛盾的是，那些工作辛苦、时间又长的人经常并不是挣钱最多的人。

paralyze ['pærəlaiz] *vt.* 使瘫痪，使麻痹；使丧失作用；使惊愕，使呆若木鸡

【例句】In May, Julie Nimmus, president of Schutt Sports in Illinois, successfully fought a lawsuit involving a football player who was paralyzed in a game while wearing a Schutt helmet.

【译文】5 月，伊利诺伊州舒特体育用品公司的总裁朱利·尼姆斯打赢了一场官司，原告是一名橄榄

球队员，他戴着舒特公司的头盔在一场比赛中
受伤瘫痪。

parental [pə'rentl]　　　　　　*a.* 父母的，父（母）亲的

partial ['pɑːʃəl]　　　　　　　*a.* 部分的，局部的；
　　　　　　　　　　　　　　　　　　偏爱的，不公平的

【例句】 The research project was only a partial success.
【译文】 那个研究课题只取得了部分成功。

participate [pɑː'tisipeit]　　　　　*vi.* 参与，参加

【搭配】 participate in 参加，参与
【例句】 Americans want to participate in all kinds of
　　　　 activities.
【译文】 美国人想参加各种各样的活动。

particle ['pɑːtikl]　　　　　　　*n.* 粒子，微粒

particularly [pə'tikjʊləli]　　　　*ad.* 特别地，尤其地

passion ['pæʃən]　　　　　　　*n.* 激情，热情；酷爱

【搭配】 have a passion for 喜爱
　　　　 be passionate for 对……热衷，对……热爱
【例句】 His skill as a player doesn't quite match his
　　　　 passion for the game.
【译文】 他的水平与他对这项游戏的酷爱程度不太相配。

patch [pætʃ]　　*n.* 小片，小块，补丁 *vt.* 补，修补

【搭配】patch up 解决（争吵、麻烦）等；修补，草草修理

patent ['pætənt]　　　　　　　　*n.* 专利权，专利品
　　　　　　　　　　　　　　vt. 取得……的专利权，请准专利
　　　['peitnt]　　　　　　　　　　　*a.* 特许的，专利的

【例句】Communications technology is generally exported from the U. S. , Europe, or Japan; the patents skills and ability to manufacture remain in the hands of a few industrialized countries.

【译文】通信技术一般是由美国、欧洲和日本出口的，专利技术技能和制造能力掌握在一些工业化国家手中。

pathogen ['pæθədʒən]　　　　　　　　　*n.* 病原体

【例句】A healthy person is given a tiny taste of a virus—flu or polio, say—that's too weak to cause illness but just enough to introduce the body to the pathogen.

【译文】一个健康的人暴露于轻微的病毒中，比如流感或小儿麻痹症，虽然病毒量太弱不会导致疾病，但足以让身体接触病原体。

pathology [pə'θɒlədʒi]　　　　　　　　　*n.* 病理学

patience ['peiʃəns]　　　　　　　　*n*. 忍耐，耐心

【搭配】run out one's patience 失去耐心
　　　　with patience 耐心地
　　　　out of patience with 对……失去耐心

【联想】patient *a*. 耐心的；*n*. 病人

payment ['peimənt]　　　　　　　*n*. 支付，付款

【搭配】in payment for 以偿付，以回报

peculiar [pi'kju:ljə]　　　*a*. 特殊的，独特的；古怪的

【搭配】be peculiar to 是……所特有的

【联想】specific to 特有的；proper to 特有的，固有的

pediatrics [ˌpi:di'ætriks]　　　　　　　*n*. 儿科

penetrate ['penitreit]　　　*v*. 穿透，渗入，看穿

【搭配】penetrate through/into 穿过，渗透

【联想】penetration *n*. 穿过，穿透

【例句】We penetrate the surface of the sculpture and pass through the crystal structure to the molecular level.

【译文】我们穿透雕塑的表面，通过晶体结构到达分子的层次。

performance [pə'fɔ:məns]　　　　　*n*. 表演，演出，执行，完成；工作情况，表现情况

【联想】perform *v*. 表演，执行

permanent [ˈpəːmənənt]　　　　　*a.* 永久的，持久的

【导学】permanent，perpetual，eternal：permanent
指永久不变的，与暂时相对；perpetual 指动
作无休止进行或状态无休止继续；eternal 表
示无始无终的，永恒的。

【例句】With tattooing, body piercing, and permanent cosmetics already well established as
fashion trends.

【译文】纹身、身体穿孔和永久性整容已经成为时尚潮流。

personality [ˌpəːsəˈnæliti]　　　　　*n.* 人格，个性

【例句】Personality in Americans is further complicated by successive waves of immigration from
various countries.

【译文】由于一波接一波外国移民的移入，美国人的性
格更复杂了。

personnel [ˌpəːsəˈnel]　　　　　*n.* 全体人员，
全体职员；人事部门

【导学】personnel 作全体员工讲时，是集合名词，所
以做主语时谓语用复数。

Day *13*

handful ['hændfl]　　　　　　　*n*. 一把，一小撮

【例句】Now a handful of researchers are warning that unpoisonous energy sources could affect the planet's climate too.

【译文】现在，一些研究人员警告说，无害能源也会影响地球的气候。

handle ['hændl]

　　　　　vt. 处理，应付；触，摸，抚弄；操纵
　　　　　n. 柄，把手，拉手

【例句】The research-integrity committee handles issues of scientific misconduct.

【译文】学术诚信委员会处理学术不端行为问题。

harass ['hærəs]　　　　*vt*. 使疲乏，困扰，反复袭击

【联想】harassment *n*. 骚扰，侵袭；烦恼

【例句】A number of black youths have complained of being harassed by the police.

【译文】许多黑人青年抱怨被警察骚扰。

harm [hɑːm]　　　　　　*n*. / *vt*. 损害，伤害，危害

【联想】 harmful *a*. 有害的；伤害的

【搭配】 come to no harm 未受到伤害
do harm to 损害，对……有害

【例句】 Breathing in other people's cigarette smoke can do real harm to your lungs.

【译文】 吸入二手烟会对你的肺有损害。

harmony ['hɑːməni]   *n*. 和谐，和睦，融洽

【联想】 harmonious *a*. 和谐的

【搭配】 in harmony with（与……）协调一致；
（与……）和睦相处

【例句】 Design criteria include harmony of colour, texture, lighting, scale, and proportion.

【译文】 设计的准则包括色彩、材质、照明、比例的协调。

hatred ['heitrid]   *n*. 憎恶，憎恨，怨恨

hazard ['hæzəd]   *n*. 危险，危害，公害

【联想】 hazardous *a*. 危险的；冒险的；危害的

【搭配】 at hazard, in danger 在危险中；at all hazards 不顾一切危险；on the hazard 受到威胁；take a hazard to do 冒险做；run the hazard / risk of doing 冒险

【例句】 Leisure centers and swimming pools were identified as potential health hazards to the very people who visit them to stay fit.

【译文】对那些为了健身的人来讲，休闲中心和游泳池被认为是潜在风险之地。

headline ['hedlain]   *n.* 大标题

【导学】辨析 heading，headline：heading 指文章定的标题、题目，也指谈话的论题、话题；headline 指报刊的大字标题、页头题目等。

heal [hiːl]   *v.* 治愈，愈合

【搭配】heal sb. of sth. 治愈某人的病

healthcare ['helθkɛə]   *n.* 医疗保健，健康护理

【例句】They are paid below the minimum wage, with no job security and no healthcare provision.

【译文】他们的工资低于最低工资，没有工作保障，也没有医疗保障。

hernia ['həːniə]   *n.* 疝

【例句】I suppose if my X-ray only showed a hernia, I must be clear.

【译文】我觉得如果我的 X 光片只显示疝气，我一定很清楚。

hippocampus [ˌhipəˈkæmpəs]   *n.* 海马体
（大脑中被认为是感情和记忆中心的部分）

【例句】Most neurons sprouting in adulthood seem to

be in the hippocampus, a structure involved in learning and memory.

【译文】大多数在成年期萌芽的神经元似乎都在海马体中，海马体是参与学习和记忆的结构。

historical [his'tɔrikəl]　　　　*a.* 历史的，有关历史的

【导学】辨析 historical，historic：historical 指历史上存在或发生过的；historic 指历史上有名的，有历史意义的。

host [həust]　　　　*n.* 主人，旅店老板；节目主持人

【导学】辨析 host，master：host 与 guest（客人）相对，即 host 招待的是 guests；master 与 servant（仆人）相对，即 master 指使的是 servant。

【搭配】a host of 一系列

【例句】Physical activity can prevent and treat a host of chronic conditions, such as heart disease, type II diabetes, and obesity.

【译文】体育活动可以预防和治疗一系列慢性疾病，如心脏病、II 型糖尿病和肥胖症。

hospitality [ˌhɔspi'tæliti]　　　　*n.* （对客人的）友好款待，好客

【导学】以-able 结尾的形容词变成名词时，往往只需将-able 变为-ability，例如：able（能……的，

有才能的）→ability（能力，才干），capable（有能力的，能干的）→capability（能力，性能，容量），changeable（可改变的）→changeability（可变性，易变性），但是请注意 hospitable（好客的，招待周到的）→hospitality（好客，殷勤）。

【例句】Thank you so much for your generous hospitality.

【译文】非常感谢您的盛情款待。

---

humane [hju:'mein]   *a*. 善良的；仁慈的；人道的

humanity [hju:'mænəti]   *n*. 人性；人类；人道；（统称）人；仁慈；人文学科

【例句】Science is supposed to benefit humanity.

【译文】科学应该造福于人类。

---

ideal [ai'diəl]   *a*. 理想的，称心如意的；唯心论的
n. 理想

【例句】Cancer vaccines would ideally be used in patients whose disease has already been diagnosed and treated with surgery, chemotherapy or radiation.

【译文】癌症疫苗最理想的应用对象是那些已经确诊且通过手术、化疗或放疗等手段治疗的患者。

---

identical [ai'dentikəl]   *a*. 相同的；同一的

【搭配】be identical with/to 和……完全相同

be identical in 在……方面相同

【导学】 辨析 be similar to，be the same as，be identical with/to：be similar to 和……相似；be the same as 和……相同；be identical with/to 和……完全相同。

【例句】 This hormone is virtually identical to the cow's own and can increase milk production by 10%～15%.

【译文】 这种激素和牛自身的几乎完全一样，能增加10%～15%的产奶量。

identify [ai'dentifai]   *vt*. 认出，鉴定；等同，打成一片

【搭配】 identify oneself with... 参加到……中去；identify...with 认为……等同于

【导学】 辨析 identify，recognize：identify 指通过某些内在的东西辨认出某人某物；recognize 指认出曾经见过或原来认识的人或物，强调通过外表认出。

【例句】 Verification of the product can be carried out in the process in order to identify variation.

【译文】 产品的验证可在运行过程中进行，以便识别变化。

identification [ai,dentifi'keiʃən]   *n*. 辨认，视为同一；证明，鉴定

【搭配】 identification card = identity card 身份证

【例句】He used a letter of introduction as identification.

【译文】他用一封介绍信作为身份的证明。

identity [ai'dentiti]　　　　　*n.* 身份；个性，特征

【例句】The police are trying to find out the identity of the woman killed in the traffic accident.

【译文】警方正在设法查清那名在交通事故中遇害的女性的身份。

ignorance ['ignərəns]　　　　*n.* 无知，愚昧

【例句】Ignorance of the law is no excuse.

【译文】不懂法律不能成为借口。

ignorant ['ignərənt]　*a.* 无知的，愚昧的；不知道的

【搭配】be ignorant of/that... 不知道，不了解

【例句】A tiny insect, trying to shake a mighty tree, is ludicrously ignorant of its own weakness.

【译文】蚍蜉撼大树，可笑不自量。

illegal [i'li:gəl]　　　　　*a.* 不合法的，非法的

【例句】Selling cigars without a license is illegal.

【译文】无执照销售雪茄烟是违法的。

illustrate ['iləstreit]　　　*vt.* 举例说明，图解

【例句】The following account by the author illustrates the difference between European and American reactions.

【译文】作者做出的下列解释说明了欧洲人和美国人在反应方面的区别。

image ['imidʒ]　　　　*n.* 像；肖像，形象；影像，图像

【联想】imagination *n.* 想象，想象力；空想，幻想

imaginable [i'mædʒinəbl]　　*a.* 可想象到的，可能的

imaginary [i'mædʒinəri] *a.* 想象的，虚构的，假想的

【例句】All the characters in the play are imaginary.

【译文】剧中所有的人物都是虚构的。

imaginative [i'mædʒinətiv] *a.* 富有想象力的，爱想象的

【导学】注意 imaginative 和 imaginary 虽然都是形容词，但它们的意思还是有区别的，imaginative 常用来形容某人富有想象力，喜欢想象，而 imaginary 多用来形容某事物或某故事是假想的，虚构的，例如：He is an imaginative writer. 他是一个富有想象力的作家。He told a story about an imaginary land. 他讲了一个关于虚构的地方的故事。

【例句】She is a very imaginative student. She's always talking about traveling to outer space.

【译文】她是一个富有想象力的学生，总是谈论关于遨游外太空的事情。

pharmaceutical [ˌfɑːmə'suːtikl] *a.* 制药的，配药的

【例句】Over the past 20 years, nearly every major pharmaceutical company has abandoned antibiotics.

【译文】在过去 20 年里，几乎所有的大型制药公司都放弃了生产抗生素。

pharmacy ['fɑːməsi]　　　*n.* 药房，药剂学，配药业，制药业

phase [feiz]　　　*n.* 阶段，时期；月相

【搭配】phase in 逐步采用；phase out 逐步停止；out of phase with 与……不协调；in phase with 与……协调

【例句】Children who were more anxious avoided eye contact during all three phases of the experiment.

【译文】更加焦虑的孩子会在试验三个阶段中都避免眼神接触。

phenomenon [fi'nɔminən]　　　*n.* 现象

【导学】phenomenon 复数形式为 phenomena。

【例句】Accordingly, they regarded dreaming as a low-level phenomenon of no great psychological interest.

【译文】因此，他们认为做梦是一种没有太大心理意义的低级现象。

physical ['fizikəl]   *a.* 物质的，有形的；身体的；自然科学的，物理的

【搭配】physical education 体育；physical strength 体力；physical constitution 体格

【例句】When a danger is psychological rather than physical, fear can force you to take self-protective measures.

【译文】当出现心理危险而非身体危险时，恐惧会迫使你采取自我保护措施。

physician [fi'ziʃən]   *n.* 内科医生

【联想】doctor 医生（一般用语）；practitioner *n.*（医生、律师等）开业者；surgeon *n.* 外科医生；dentist *n.* 牙医

【例句】There is no doubt that the virtual visit is a fundamental alteration to the patient-physician encounter.

【译文】毫无疑问，虚拟就诊是对医患关系的根本改变。

physicist ['fizisist]   *n.* 物理学家

plague [pleig]   *n.* 瘟疫；麻烦，苦恼，灾祸
vt. 折磨，使苦恼

【例句】They all seemed to be plagued by annoying technical issues.

【译文】他们似乎都被恼人的技术问题所困扰。

pleased [pli:zd]   *a*. 高兴的，满足的

politician [pɔli'tiʃən]   *n*. 政治家，政客
【联想】statesman *n*. 政治家（含褒义）

politics ['pɔlitiks]   *n*. 政治；政见，政纲

pollute [pə'lu:t]   *vt*. 污染，玷污
【联想】pollution *n*. 污染；pollutant *n*. 污染物质
【例句】Integrated thinking is also needed to mitigate urban air pollution.
【译文】缓解城市空气污染也需要综合思维。

populate ['pɔpjuleit]   *v*. 使人民居住，移民
【联想】population *n*. 人口
     repopulate *vt*. 重新住人；种群恢复
【例句】Once repopulated with healthy cells, these livers lived in culture for 10 days.
【译文】一旦用健康细胞重新填充，这些肝脏可以在培养物中存活10天。

portable ['pɔ:təbl]   *a*. 轻便的，手提（式）的
【例句】The documents have been typed into a portable computer.
【译文】文件已经被输入到一台便携式电脑里了。

portrait ['pɔ:trit]   *n*. 肖像，画像

potential [pə'tenʃ(ə)l]　　　　　*a*. 潜在的，可能的

　　　　　　　　　　　　　　　　n. 潜力，潜能

【例句】 It's much to be regretted that he died so young, his potential unfulfilled.

【译文】 他才华未展，英年早逝，十分令人惋惜。

practicable ['præktikəbl]　　　　　*a*. 能实行的，

　　　　　　　　　　　　　　行得通的，可以实行的

【联想】 practically *ad*. 实际上；几乎

practitioner [præk'tiʃənə]　　　　*n*. 开业医生；律师

precaution [pri'kɔːʃən]　　　　*n*. 预防，留心，警戒

　　　　　　　　　　　　　　　vt. 预告，警告

【例句】 Our first priority is to take every precaution to protect our citizens at home and around the world from further attacks.

【译文】 我们首要任务是采取一切预防措施，以保证我们的公民不论是在家还是在世界上的其他地方都不再受到袭击。

pregnant ['pregnənt]　　　　　　*a*. 怀孕的

【联想】 pregnancy *n*. 怀孕，怀孕期

premature [ˌpremə'tjuə]　　　　*a*. 未成熟的，早熟的

【例句】 Vergil is still recovering from premature birth.

【译文】 维吉尔仍有早产后遗症，正在恢复。

preliminary [priˈliminəri]　　　　*a*. 预备的，初步的

【例句】In the normal grant system, preliminary data requirements make it hard to start new directions in research.

【译文】在平常的资金资助体系中，对研究基础的数据要求使其很难开创研究的新方向。

prenatal [ˌpriːˈneitl]　　　　　　　　*a*. 孕期的

【例句】Prenatal caffeine consumption may have more detrimental long-term effects on liver development.

【译文】产前摄入咖啡因可能会对肝脏发育产生更有害的长期影响。

preparation [ˌprepəˈreiʃən]　　　*n*. 准备，预备；制备品，制剂

【搭配】make preparations for 为……做准备；in preparation 在准备中；in preparation for 作为……的准备

prescribe [prisˈkraib]　*vt*. 开处方，开药；规定，指示

【搭配】prescribe for 为……开处方

【例句】The doctor prescribed his patient a receipt.

【译文】医生给病人开了一张药方。

presence [ˈprezns]　　　　　　*n*. 出席，在场；存在

【搭配】in the presence of sb. 当着某人的面，有某人

在场；presence of mind 镇定自若

presentation [ˌprezn'teiʃən]　　*n*. 介绍，陈述；表现形式

presumably [pri'zju:məbli]　　　*ad*. 推测起来，大概

prevail [pri'veil]　　　*vi*. 取胜，占优势；流行，盛行

【搭配】 prevail over/against 战胜，压倒；prevail in/
among 流行，普遍存在；prevail on/upon sb.
to do sth. 劝说某人做某事

【例句】 Nothing is so uncertain as the fashion market
where one style prevails over another.

【译文】 没有什么事情比时尚市场更不确定了，一种风
格更胜另一种风格。

prevalent ['prevələnt]　　　　*n*. 流行的，普遍的

【导学】 近义词：widespread, accepted, common,
prevailing

【例句】 Diabetes is one of the most prevalent and
potentially dangerous diseases in the world.

【译文】 糖尿病是世界上最流行和有潜在危险的疾病
之一。

primary ['praiməri]　　*a*. 首要的，主要的，基本的；
最初的，初级的

【例句】 Building trust is a primary goal.

【译文】建立信任是首要（primary：essential）目标。

procedure [prəˈsiːdʒə]　　　　　　　　　*n*. 程序

【例句】The procedure was even successful in several patients whose burn injuries had occurred years earlier and who had already undergone surgery.

【译文】甚至几位早年眼灼伤并且已接受过手术的患者，治疗都取得了成功。

proceed [prəˈsiːd]　　　　　　　　　*vi*. 继续进行

【搭配】proceed to do sth. 继续做（另一件事）
proceed with sth. 继续进行

【例句】Once your PIN has been reset，you may proceed to create a new PIN.

【译文】一旦您的 PIN 被重新设置，您就可以继续创建新的 PIN。

profession [prəˈfeʃən]　　　　　*n*. 职业，自由职业

【搭配】by profession 在职业上，就职业而言

professional [prəˈfeʃənl]　　　*a*. 职业的，专门的
　　　　　　　　　　　　　　　　　　　n. 专业人员

【例句】He has just turned professional.

【译文】他刚成为专业人士。

Day *14*

immigrant ['imigrənt]   *n.* 移民，侨民 *a.* 移民的

【导学】辨析 immigrant，emigrant：immigrant 指的是来自国外的移民，指为了永久居住而从别国到居住国的人；emigrant 指的是离开国家或地区到别国永久居住的人。

【例句】A family approach to health care is recommended for immigrant groups.

【译文】建议移民群体采用家庭医疗方式。

impact ['impækt]   *n.* 影响，作用；冲击，碰撞

【搭配】have an impact on sth. 对……的影响

【例句】On the other hand, the impact of environmental influences is still largely a mystery.

【译文】另一方面，环境影响的程度在很大程度上仍然是一个谜。

impair [im'pɛə]   *v.* 损害，损伤，削弱

【导学】近义词：spoil，injure，hurt，damage，destroy；diminish，undermine，reduce，weaken

【例句】Having too much caffeine during pregnancy may impair baby's liver development.

【译文】孕期摄入过多咖啡因会伤害胎儿的肝脏发育。

imperative [im'perətiv]　*a.* 必要的，紧急的，极重的；命令的 *n.* 必要的事，必须完成的事；祈使语气

【例句】Military orders are imperative and cannot be disobeyed.

【译文】军令是强制性的，必须遵守。

impatient [im'peiʃənt]　　　*a.* 不耐烦的，急躁的

【搭配】be impatient of 对……不耐烦，不能忍受

be impatient for/to do 急切

implicate ['implikeit]　*vt.* 牵连；牵涉，涉及（某人）；表明（或意指）……是起因

【例句】He tried to avoid saying anything that would implicate him further.

【译文】他尽力避免说出任何会进一步牵连他的事情。

inadequate [in'ædikwət]　　　　*a.* 不充分的；不足的；不够的；不胜任的

【例句】The supplies of food are inadequate to meet the needs.

【译文】食物供给还不能充分满足需求。

incidence ['insidəns]　　　　　　*n.* 发生（率）

【例句】At present，it is not possible to confirm or to

refute the suggestion that there is a causal relationship between the amount of fat we eat and the incidence of heart attacks.

【译文】目前我们很难决定应该赞成还是反驳这种观点，即脂肪的摄入量和心脏发病率之间存在着因果关系。

incidentally [insi'dentəli]   ad. 附带提及地，顺便地

【导学】有些副词用来表示评价一件事，或说明一种状态，可以单独放在句首，除 incidentally 以外，常见的还有：fortunately 幸运的是，unfortunately 不幸地，luckily 幸运地，generally（或 generally speaking）一般说来。

【例句】I must go now. Incidentally, if you want that book I'll bring it next time.

【译文】我现在该走了。顺便提一句，如果你要那本书，我下次带来。

incident ['insidənt]   n. 事件，政治事件，事变

【例句】Incidents of misconduct in the news tend to describe the most serious violations of scientific standards, such as plagiarism for fabricating data.

【译文】新闻中的不当行为事件往往描述最严重的学术违规行为，例如伪造数据的剽窃行为。

incline [in'klain]　　　　*v*. 使倾向，使倾斜，使偏向

　　　　　　　　　　　　　n. 斜坡，斜面

【搭配】 incline to/towards sth. 有……的倾向；be inclined to do sth. 想做某事，有……的趋势

incorporate [in'kɔ:pəreit]　　　　*vt*. 结合，合并，

使加入，收编 *vi*. 合并，混合

【例句】 We will incorporate your suggestion in the new plan.

【译文】 我们将把你的建议纳入新计划。

increasingly [in'kri:siŋli]　　　*ad*. 日益地，越来越多地

【例句】 The international situation has been growing increasingly difficult for the last few years.

【译文】 最近几年国际形势越来越严峻。

indicate ['indikeit]　　　　　*vt*. 指示，表示；暗示

【联想】 indication *n*. 指示，表示；暗示

【例句】 Overall our analysis indicated that women may be more vulnerable to the effects of smoking.

【译文】 总体而言，我们的分析表明，女性可能更容易受到吸烟的影响。

indicator ['indikeitə]　　　　　　*n*. 指示器，指示剂；

[计算机] 指示符

【例句】Body shape is known to be a risk indicator for heart disease and diabetes.

【译文】众所周知，体型是心脏病和糖尿病的危险指标。

individual [ˌindiˈvidjuəl] *a.* 个别的，单独的；独特的
n. 个人，个体

【导学】辨析 individual，personal，private：individual 意为"独立于他人的，各个的，个别的"，与 general（普遍的）和 collective（集体的）相对；personal 意思是"个人的，亲自的"；private 意为"私人的，秘密的"，与 public（公共的，共有的）相对。

【例句】The other reason to oppose the death penalty is largely a matter of individual conscience and belief.

【译文】另外一个反对死刑的原因主要是个人良知和信仰的问题。

industrial [inˈdʌstriəl] *a.* 工业的；产业的

【导学】辨析 industrial，industrious：industrial 意为"工业的，产业的"；industrious 意为"勤劳的，勤奋的"。

inevitable [inˈevitəbl] *a.* 不可避免的，必然的

【例句】It is inevitable that some changes will take

place.

【译文】有些变化将要发生，不可避免。

infant ['infənt]   *n.* 婴儿，幼儿

inflame [in'fleim]   *vt.* 使（局势）恶化；激起……
的强烈感情

inflation [in'fleiʃən]   *n.* 通货膨胀

【例句】If the gain of profit is solely due to rising
energy prices, then inflation should be
subsided when energy price wears off.

【译文】如果收益仅仅来自能源价格上涨，那么当能源
价格下调时，通货膨胀应该会逐渐消退。

influence ['influəns]   *n.* 势力，权势
vt. /n. 影响，感化

【搭配】have influence on/upon 影响

【联想】influential *a.* 有影响的，有势力的

【例句】It also has some negative influence.

【译文】这也有一些负面影响。

infrastructure ['infrəstrʌktʃə(r)]
n. 基础设施，基础建设

inform [in'fɔːm] *vt.* 通知，告诉，报告；告发，告密

【搭配】inform sb. of sth. 把某事告知某人

inform against/on sb. 告发，检举某人

【导学】辨析 inform，notify：inform 意为"告诉，通知"，强调直接把任何种类的事实或知识告诉或传递给某人；notify 意为"通知"，指用官方公告或正式通知书将所应该或需要知道的事告诉某人，含有情况紧急，需要立刻采取行动或及早答复的意思。

【例句】It's time to use this fusion of biology and sociology to inform public policy.

【译文】是时候利用生物学和社会学的融合来指导公共政策了。

initial [i'niʃəl]　　　　*a.* 最初的，开头的 *n.* 首字母

【导学】辨析 initial，original，primary，primitive：initial 意为"最初的，开始的"，强调处于事物的起始阶段的，开头的，也可指位于开头地方的；original 意为"最早的，最先的"，强调处于事物的起始阶段的，按顺序应是首位的，也可指原始的、原件的，即非仿造的东西；primary 指在时间、顺序或发展上领先的（第一的、基本的、主要的）；primitive 指处于人类生命或事物发展的早期阶段的、原始的。

initiate [i'niʃieit]　　　　　*vt.* 开始，创始，发动；
启蒙，使入门；引入，正式介绍

【搭配】 be initiated into 正式加入；initiate sb. into sth. 准许或介绍某人加入某团体，把某事传授给某人

【例句】 We should initiate a new social custom.

【译文】 我们要开创社会新风尚。

initiative [i'niʃiətiv]　　　　　*n.* 创始，首创精神；
决断的能力；主动性 *a.* 起始的，初步的

【例句】 Two decade ago a woman who shook hands with men on her own initiative was usually viewed as too forward.

【译文】 20年前，主动和男性握手的女性通常被认为是非常前卫的人。

innocent ['inəsnt]　　　　　*a.* 无罪的，清白的；
无害的；天真的，单纯的

【搭配】 be innocent of 无意识的，无……罪的

【联想】 be guilty of 有……罪

【例句】 The workers were merely absent-minded and sometimes made innocent errors.

【译文】 工人们只是心不在焉，有时犯了无心之过。

innovation [ˌinəu'veiʃən]　　　　　*n.* 创新，改革

【例句】Given this optimistic approach to technological innovation，the American worker took readily to that special kind of nonverbal thinking required in mechanical technology.

【译文】有了这种对技术革新的乐观态度，美国工人很快便习惯了机械技术所需要的非语言的思维方式。

intact [in'tækt]　　　　　　*a*. 未经触动的，原封不动的，完整无损的

【例句】The task then is to find proxies（普代物）for key traits and behaviors that have stayed intact over millennia.

【译文】人们的任务就是找到这些千年不变的关键特质和行为的替代物。

intake ['inteik]　　*n*. 摄入；（食物、饮料等的）摄取量，吸入量；（一定时期内）纳入的人数；吸收

【例句】In young and middle-aged adults，restricting calorie intake can have an impact on their health.

【译文】年轻人和中年人限制热量摄入会对健康产生影响。

insomnia [in'sɔmniə]　　　　　　　*n*. 失眠症

【例句】It can grow things like feeling anxious，or having insomnia，very dizzy，and having nausea.

【译文】它会产生焦虑、失眠、头晕和恶心等症状。

inspect [in'spekt]　　　　　　　*vt.* 检查，调查，视察

【例句】All factories and mines are inspected by government officials.

【译文】所有工厂和矿井都要接受政府官员的视察。

install [in'stɔːl]　　　　　　　　　　*vt.* 安装，设置

【联想】installation *n.* 安装，设置

installment [in'stɔːlmənt]　　　　*n.* 分期付款；
　　　　　　　　　　　　　　　　　（连载的）一部分，一期

【例句】We pay for our holidays in installment of $ 50 a month.

【译文】我们以每月50美元分期付款的方式度假。

instance ['instəns]　　　　　　　　*n.* 例证，实例

【搭配】for instance 举例说，比如

instant ['instənt]　*n.* 瞬间，时刻 *a.* 立即的，立刻的；
　　　　　　紧急的，迫切的；（食品）速溶的，方便的

【搭配】on the instant 立即；the instant（that）一……
　　　就（引导时间状语从句）

【例句】You see the lightening the instant it happens, but you hear the thunder later.

【译文】 你可以在闪电发生的瞬间立刻看见它，但要稍后才能听到雷声。

insurance [in'ʃuərəns] *n.* 保险，保险费

【例句】 After the robbery, the shop installed a sophisticated alarm system as an insurance against further losses.

【译文】 抢劫发生以后，商店装了一套精密复杂的警报系统，以防止进一步的损失。

insure [in'ʃuə] *vi.* 保险，替……保险；保证

【搭配】 insure sb. /sth. against 给某人或某物保险以防

【联想】 assure sb. of sth. /that 使某人确信；convince sb. of sth., ensure sth. 确保某事；make sure that 保证

【例句】 It is advisable to insure your life against accident.

【译文】 最好参加人寿保险，以防意外。

integrity [in'tegriti] *n.* 诚实，正直，完整

【例句】 They have always regarded man of integrity and fairness as a reliable friend.

【译文】 他们一直认为诚实、正直的人是可信赖的朋友。

integrate ['intigreit] *vt.* 使结合，使一体化

【搭配】 integrate...with... 把……与……相结合
integrate...into 使……并入

【例句】Many suggestions are need to integrate the plan.

【译文】需要许多建议使计划更加完整。

promote [prə'məut]　　　　　　　*vt*. 提升，晋升；促进，增进，助长

【例句】They have greatly promoted American culture, and improved the living standards of the whole American people.

【译文】他们极大促进了美国文化的发展，提高了所有美国人的生活水平。

proof [pru:f]　　　　　　　　　　*n*. 证据，证明

property ['prɔpəti]　　　　*n*. 财产，所/物；性质，特性

【搭配】movable/personal property 动产
　　　　real property 不动产

proportion [prə'pɔ:ʃən]　　　　　*n*. 部分，份额；比例，比重；均衡，相称

【搭配】in proportion to 与……成比例
　　　　out of proportion to 与……不成比例

【例句】Gradually raise the proportion of the tertiary industry in the national economy.

【译文】逐步提高第三产业在国民经济中的比重。

proposal [prə'pəʊzəl]　　　　　　*n.* 提议，建议；求婚

【导学】在 proposal 后的同位语从句和表语从句中，谓语用虚拟语气。

辨析 proposal，suggest：proposal 意为"提议，忠告"，指正式或通过一定程序或途径而提出的建议；suggest 意为"建议"，指所提建议不一定正确，仅供对方参考。

propose [prə'pəʊz]　　　　　　*vt.* 提议，建议；求婚

【搭配】propose doing 建议做某事；propose to do 打算做某事；propose to sb. 向某人求婚

【导学】propose 的宾语从句中谓语用虚拟语气。

prostate ['prɒsteit]　　　　　　*n.* 前列腺

psychiatrist [saɪ'kaɪətrɪst] *n.* 精神病医师，精神病学家

【导学】psychic 通灵的人；psychiatry 精神病学；psycho 精神病患者；psychology 心理学；psychologist 心理学家人 = 试图用精神分析治疗病人的人 = psychiatrist 精神病学家，精神病医师

【例句】"The material on immigrant health shocked me when we first reviewed it." says panel member Arthus M. Kleinman，a psychiatrist and anthropologist at Harvard Medical School in Boston.

【译文】"当我们第一次审阅移民健康的资料时，我感到十分震惊。"审阅委员会的成员亚瑟 M. 克莱曼说。他是波士顿哈佛医学院的精神病学家和人类学家。

psychological [ˌsaikə'lɔdʒikəl]　　*a*. 心理（上）的，心理学的

【联想】psychology *n*. 心理学；psychologist *n*. 心理学家

【例句】Freud's psychological map may have been flawed in many ways，but it also happens to be the most coherent and meaningful theory of the mind.

【译文】弗洛伊德的心理图谱可能在很多方面都有缺陷，但它也恰好是最连贯的、最有意义的精神理论。

publicity [pʌb'lisiti]　*n*. 众所周知，闻名；宣传，广告

【联想】publication *n*. 发表，公布，出版

【例句】Pasteur received wide acclaim and much favorable publicity.

【译文】巴斯德获得了广泛的赞誉和好评。

purchase ['pəːtʃəs]　*n*. 购买；购买的东西 *vt*. 购买

quarter ['kwɔːtə]　　　*n*. 四分之一；一刻钟；季度

qualify [ˈkwɒlifai]　　*vt.* 取得资格，使合格，使胜任

【搭配】qualify as 有条件成为

【联想】qualification *n.* 资格，条件，限制，限定

【例句】Heat stroke is a medical emergency that demands immediate intervention from qualified medical personnel.

【译文】中暑是一种医疗紧急情况，需要合格的医务人员即时干预。

Day 14

Day 15

intellect ['intilekt]　　　　　*n*. 理智，智力；有才智的人

intellectual [inti'lektʃuəl]　　　　　*n*. 知识分子
　　　　　a. 智力的；显示智力的，能发挥才智的

【例句】More legislation is needed to protect the intellectual property rights of the patent.

【译文】需要更多立法保护专利知识产权。

intelligent [in'telidʒənt]　　　　　*a*. 聪明的，理智的

【联想】intelligence *n*. 智力；理解力；情报，消息，报道

【例句】He was intelligent enough to understand my questions from the gestures I made.

【译文】他非常聪明，能根据我的手势明白我的问题。

intelligible [in'telidʒəbl]　　　　　*a*. 可以理解的，易领悟的，清晰的

【联想】名词 intelligence 智慧，智力，智商 intelligible = intellig + ible（able）需要智慧才能理解的；intelligent 智慧的，聪明的

【例句】This report would be intelligible only to an

expert in computing.

【译文】 只有计算机专家才能明白这个报道。

intend [in'tend] *vt*. 想要，打算，企图

【搭配】 intend to do sth. 打算做某事
be intended as/for 原意要，意指……

intense [in'tens] *a*. 强烈的，激烈的，热烈的

【例句】 In the Arctic，the effects of climate change are most intense.

【译文】 北极圈内，气候变化的影响最为强烈。

intensive [in'tensiv] *a*. 加强的，密集的；精工细作的

【导学】 辨析 intense，intensive：intense 意为"激烈的，强烈的"，如 intense competition（激烈的竞争）；intensive 意为"集中的，加强的"，如 intensive reading（精读）。

【例句】 The patient's health failed to such an extent that he was put into intensive care.

【译文】 这名病人的病情恶化得相当严重，因此对他进行了重病特别护理。

intention [in'tenʃən] *n*. 意图，意向，目的

【例句】 She had clearly no intention of doing any work，although she was very well paid.

【译文】 她明显不打算干任何工作，尽管她的工资待遇很不错。

interdiscipline [ˌintə'disiplin]   *n*. 交叉学科

【联想】interdisciplinary *a*. 交叉学科的

【联想】interdisciplinary *a*. 跨学科的

【例句】Much of the most important research is now interdisciplinary in nature.

【译文】很多最重要的研究在本质上都是跨学科的。

interface ['intə(ː)feis]   , *n*. 界面，接口

【例句】Much of the intellectual action in our society today lies at the interfaces between traditional disciplines.

【译文】今天，我们社会中的许多智力活动都发生在传统学科之间的连接处。

interactive [ˌintər'æktiv]   *a*. 相互作用的，相互影响的

internal [in'təːnl]   *a*. 内的，内部的；国内的，内政的

【例句】He suffered internal injuries in the accident.

【译文】他在这次事故中受了内伤。

interpret [in'təːprit]   *vt*. 解释；说明；口译；翻译

【联想】interpretation *n*. 解释，阐明

【导学】辨析 translate，interpret：translate 指口头或笔头翻译；interpret 仅指口头翻译。

【例句】I interpreted his answer as a refusal.

【译文】我把他的回答理解为拒绝。

interrupt [ˌɪntəˈrʌpt]　　*vt.* 打断，打扰；断绝，中断

【导学】 辨析 bankrupt，corrupt，interrupt：bankrupt 意为"破产的"；corrupt 意为"贪污的"；interrupt 意为"中断，打断"。

interval [ˈɪntəvəl]　　　　　　*n.* 间隔，间歇

【搭配】 at intervals 有时，不时，时时；at an interval of 间隔/间距（多长时间/多远）

intimate [ˈɪntɪmɪt]　　　　　*a.* 亲密的，密切的

【例句】 These week-long meetings are designed to promote intimate, informal discussions of frontier science.

【译文】 这些长达一周的会议旨在促进对前沿科学非正式的密切讨论。

invade [ɪnˈveɪd]　　　　　*vt.* 侵入，侵略，侵害

【联想】 invasion *n.* 侵入，侵略

【例句】 She got annoyed when her colleague invaded her privacy.

【译文】 当同事侵犯她的隐私时，她很生气。

invalid [ɪnˈvælɪd]　　*a.* （指法律上）无效的，作废的；无可靠根据的，站不住脚的 *n.* (the) 病弱者，残疾者

【例句】 Your license has been invalid.

195

【译文】你的执照已经作废了。

investigate [in'vestigeit]　　　　　v. 调查，调研

【搭配】investigate (into) sth. 对某事进行调查

【例句】There's an imbalance between our ability to investigate the genome and the environment.

【译文】人们研究环境因素的能力和研究基因组的能力存在差距。

irradiate [i'reidieit]　　　　　v. 照耀，辐射，
(使) 灿烂，(使) 明亮

【例句】He rapidly became irradiated with his own power in the team.

【译文】他的能力让他很快在团队中脱颖而出。

irrational [i'ræʃənl]　　　　　a. 不合理的；
不合逻辑的；没有道理的

【例句】She has an irrational dread of hospitals.

【译文】她莫名其妙地害怕医院。

ironic(al) [ai'rɔnik(əl)]　　　　　a. 讽刺的，冷嘲的

irony ['airəni]　　　　　n. 反话，讽刺

【例句】The irony of the historian's craft is that its practitioners always know that their efforts are but contributions to an unending process.

【译文】 对历史学家技艺具有讽刺意味的是，参与实践者总是明白，他们的努力只是对一个无穷的过程的小小奉献。

isolate [ˈaisəleit]   *vt.* 隔离，孤立

【联想】 isolation *n.* 隔离，孤立
【搭配】 be isolated from 脱离，被隔离，被孤立
【例句】 Several villages have been isolated by the floods.
【译文】 洪水使好几座村庄与外界隔绝了。

obituary [əˈbitʃuəri]   *n.* 讣告 *a.* 死亡的，讣告的

obligation [ˌɔbliˈgeiʃən]   *n.* 义务；职责；责任

【搭配】 be under no/an obligation（to do sth.）（没）有义务（做某事）
【例句】 Parents have a legal obligation to ensure that their children are provided with efficient education suitable to their age.
【译文】 父母在法律上有义务确保他们的孩子可以获得适合他们年龄的有效教育。

observe [əbˈzəːv]   *vt.* 观察，注意到，看到
                                遵守，奉行；说，评论

【联想】 observer *n.* 观察员

observation *n.* 观察，监视，评论，意见

【搭配】 observe on/upon 评论

【例句】 The scientist continues to experiment and observe until the theories are proved.

【译文】 这个科学家继续做实验并进行观察，直到这些理论被证明。

obstacle ['ɔbstəkl]　　　　　　　　　　*n.* 障碍

【例句】 Materialism and individualism in American society are the biggest obstacles.

【译文】 唯物主义和个人主义是美国社会最大的障碍。

obtain [əb'tein]　　　　　　　　　*vt.* 获得，得到

occasion [ə'keiʒən] *n.* 场合；大事，节日；时机，机会

【搭配】 on occasion 有时，偶尔

　　　　on the occasion of... 在……的时候

【联想】 occasional *a.* 偶然的，不时的

occupation [ˌɔkju'peiʃən]　　　　　　*n.* 占领，职业

【联想】 occupational *a.* 职业的

occupy ['ɔkjupai]　　　　　　　　*vt.* 占，占领，占据；
　　　　　　　　　　　　　　　　　使忙碌，使从事

【搭配】 occupy oneself in doing sth. /with sth. 忙着

（做某事）；忙（于某事）；be occupied with/
in 忙于

【例句】 You were signaled forward to occupy the seat
opposite him.

【译文】 有人暗示你向前去占他对面的座位。

operational [ˌɔpəˈreiʃnəl]　　　　　a. 操作的，运作的

operator [ˈɔpəreitə]　　n. 操作人员；（电话）接线员

orphan [ˈɔːfən]　　　　　n. 孤儿 a. 无父母的

opponent [əˈpəunənt]　　　　　　n. 对手，敌手

【例句】 We cannot look down upon our opponent，
who is an experienced swimmer.

【译文】 我们不能轻视我们的对手，他是一名有经验的
游泳选手。

opportunity [ˌɔpəˈtjuːniti]　　　　　　　n. 机会

【例句】 About 60 percent of American adults nap
when given the opportunity.

【译文】 大约60%的美国成年人在有机会的时候会小睡
一下。

oppose [əˈpəuz]　　　　　　vt. 反对，反抗

【搭配】 be opposed to sth. /doing sth. 反对

【例句】 But they won't think this way; they will oppose us stubbornly.

【译文】 可是，他们不会这样想，他们会坚决反对我们。

optical [ˈɒptikəl]　　　　*a*. 光学的，光的；视觉的，视力的

oral [ˈɔːrəl]　　　　　　　　　　　*a*. 口的；口头的

【例句】 This drug is available for both oral and parenteral administration.

【译文】 本药可供口服或注射用。

organ [ˈɔːɡən]　　　　　　　　　*n*. 机构；器官；风琴

【联想】 organism *n*. 组织，机体

【例句】 The FBI is an organ of the Justice Department.

【译文】 联邦调查局是司法部的一个机构。

organic [ɔːˈɡænik]　　　　　　　　*a*. 有机体的，器官的

【搭配】 organic food 有机食物

organize [ˈɔːɡənaiz]　　　　　　　　*vt*. 组织，组编

【联想】 organization *n*. 组织，体制；团体，机构

origin [ˈɒridʒin]　　　　*n*. 起源，由来；出身，血统

【导学】 辨析 origin，root，source：origin 指事物的起源或者开端，着重于其发生的最早的时间或最初的地点，常表示某种历史文化现象、

风俗习惯的起源，也可指人的门第或血统；root 常译为"根源，起因"，强调导致某事物最终出现的最根本的、最重要的原因，由此所产生的现象或事物常成为一种外观的产物；source 指河流或泉水的发源地，也是非物质的或无形的东西的出处或起源，常指情况或信息的来源、出处。

original [əˈridʒənəl]　　　　*a.* 最初的，原始的，原文的；新颖的，有独创性的

【例句】Internet was originally designed to promote education.

【译文】互联网最初是为普及教育而设计的。

originate [əˈridʒineit]　*vt.* 引起，发明，发起，创办　　　　　　　　　　　　*vi.* 起源，发生

【搭配】originate from/in/with 产生于

outbreak [ˈautbreik]　　　*n.* （战争、情感、火山等的）爆发；（疾病、虫害等的）突然发生

【例句】During the acute phase of the outbreak, it is necessary to keep suspects at special risk under observation.

【译文】在爆发的急剧阶段，必须将面临特殊威胁的疑似病例置于监视之下。

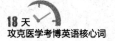
overall [ˈəuvərɔːl]   *a.* 全面的，综合的

【例句】 Promoting practice guidelines might have a much bigger effect on the overall health of Americans.

【译文】 推广实践指南可能会对美国人的整体健康产生更大的影响。

Day *16*

label [ˈleibl]　　*n.* 标签，标记 *v.* 贴标签，把……称为

【例句】Is that label accurate? Is it intolerant to challenge another's opinion? It depends on what definition of opinion you have in mind.

【译文】那个商标准确吗？去挑战他人的观点是否是偏执的呢？它完全取决于你心里对意见的定义。

laboratory [ləˈbɒrətəri]　　　　　　*n.* 实验室，研究室

largely [ˈlɑːdʒli]　　*ad.* 大部分，基本上；大规模地

【例句】These gases are caused largely by livestock waste and synthetic fertilizers.

【译文】这些气体主要是由牲畜粪便和合成肥料产生的。

laser [ˈleizə]　　　　　　　　　　　　　*n.* 激光

launch [lɔːntʃ]　　*vt.* 发射；下水；开始，发起
　　　　　　　　　　　　　n. 发射；下水

【搭配】launch an attack on/against 对……发动进攻

【例句】Meanwhile, several biotech companies are launching trials combining neoantigen vaccines and checkpoint inhibitors for various cancers.

【译文】与此同时，几家生物技术公司正在开展新抗原疫苗和检查点抑制剂联合治疗各种癌症的试验。

lawsuit ['lɔːsjuːt]   *n.* 诉讼

leader ['liːdə]   *n.* 领袖，领导者

leadership ['liːdəʃip]   *n.* 领导

【搭配】under the leadership of 在……的领导下

leading ['liːdiŋ]   *a.* 指导的，领导的；领先的；第……位的，最主要的

【例句】Liver disease is the 12th leading cause of death in the U. S.

【译文】肝病致死率在美国位居第 12 位。

learned ['ləːnid]   *a.* 有学问的，博学的

legacy ['legəsi]   *n.* 遗产；遗赠财物；遗留；后遗症

【例句】Future generations will be left with a legacy of pollution and destruction.

【译文】留给子孙后代的将是环境的污染与破坏。

legal ['liːgl]   *a.* 合法的；法律的；与法律有关的；法律允许的；法律要求的

【例句】 The legal system is not doing much to dispel that notion.

【译文】 法律体系在消除这种观念方面做得并不多。

legislation [ˌledʒisˈleiʃən]　*n*. 立法，法律的制定 /通过

【例句】 More legislation is needed to protect the intellectual property rights of the patent.

【译文】 需要更多的立法来保护专利的知识产权。

legislative [ˈledʒisleitiv]　*a*. 立法的，立法机关的
　　　　　　　　　　　　　　　　n. 立法机关

legislator [ˈledʒisleitə]　*n*. 立法者

lethal [ˈliːθəl]　*a*. 致命的，毁灭性的，有效的
　　　　　　　　　n. 基因异常，致死基因

【例句】 It has been proved that the chemical is lethal to rats but safe for cattle.

【译文】 经证实，这种化学药品对于鼠类是致命的，但对家禽无害。

leukemia [luːˈkiːmiə]　*n*. 白血病

liable [ˈlaiəbl]　*a*. 有……倾向性，易于；有偿付责任的

【搭配】 be liable to 易于；be liable for 对……有责任

【例句】 A child can be born weak or liable to serious illness as a result of radiation.

【译文】 因为辐射，孩子刚刚出生就可能很虚弱或者易于罹患严重的疾病。

liability [ˌlaiəˈbiliti]　　　　　　n. 责任，义务；
　　　　　　　　　　　　　　　　　(pl.) 债务，负债

【搭配】 a liability for 是……的责任
　　　　a liability to do 做……的责任

【例句】 A few common misconceptions：Beauty is only skin-deep. One's physical assets and liabilities don't count all that much in a managerial career.

【译文】 有一些普遍的错误看法：美丽只是表面的。在管理职业生涯中，一个人外表的美丑并不意味着全部。

limitation [ˌlimiˈteiʃən]　　　n. 缺陷，限额，限制

【例句】 With all its advantages，the computer is by no means without its limitations.

【译文】 尽管计算机有很多优点，但它也绝不是没有缺陷的。

limited [ˈlimitid]　　　　　　a. 被限定的，有限的

link [liŋk]　　　v. 连接，联系 n. 环，链环；联系

liquid [ˈlikwid]　　　　　　　　　　　n. 液体
　　　　a. 液体的，液态的；流动的；可兑换成现金的

【联想】 solid *n*. 固体；gas *n*. 气体

liquor ['likə]   *n*. 酒

literary ['litərəri] *a*. 文学的；精通文学的，从事写作的

【联想】 literal *a*. 字面的，正确的，乏味的
       literate *a*. 有文化的，识字的

literature ['litəritʃə]   *n*. 文学，文学作品；文献

【搭配】 contemporary literature 当代文学
       light literature 通俗文学

loan [ləun]   *n*. 贷款 *v*. /*n*. 借出

【搭配】 on loan 暂借的（地）

lubricate ['lu:brikeit]   *vt*. 润滑，加润滑油

【联想】 lubrication *n*. 润滑；lubricator *n*. 润滑物；
       加油工

【例句】 You should lubricate the wheels of your bicycle
       once a month.

【译文】 你应该每个月给自行车轮子加一次润滑油。

local ['ləukəl]   *a*. 地方的，当地的；局部的

locate [ləu'keit]   *vt*. 找出，查出；设置在，位于
                          vi. 定居下来

【搭配】 be located in/by/on 坐落于，位于

【例句】Early settlers located where there was water.

【译文】早期的移民者在有水的地方定居下来。

location [ləuˈkeiʃən]　　*n*.位置，地点；定位，测量

loyal [ˈlɔiəl]　　　　　　*a*.忠诚的，忠贞的

loyalty [ˈlɔiəlti]　　　　　*n*.忠诚，忠心

【例句】As a demanding boss, he expected total loyalty and dedication from his employees.

【译文】他是个苛刻的老板，要求手下的人对他忠心耿耿、鞠躬尽瘁。

nasty [ˈnæsti]　*a*.极令人不快的；很脏的；危险的

【导学】和该词意思相反的是 pleasant（愉快的，可爱的）。

【例句】Since the dawn of human ingenuity, people have devised ever more cunning tools to cope with work that is dangerous, boring, burdensome, or just plain nasty.

【译文】自从人类灵智开发以来，就一直在设计越来越精巧的工具，去应付那些危险、枯燥、繁重或实在不堪忍受的各种劳动。

nausea [ˈnɔːziə]　　　　*n*.恶心，作呕，反胃

nearby [ˈniəbai]　*a*./*ad*.附近 *prep*.在……附近

【导学】 nearby 既可以做前置定语，也可以做后置定语。辨析 nearby，near：nearby 指空间，不指时间；near 可指时间和空间。

necessarily [nesi'serili]　　*ad.* 必然，必定；当然

【搭配】 not necessarily 未必（表部分否定）

necessity [ni'sesiti]　　*n.* 必要性，必然性；必需品

【搭配】 of necessity 无法避免地，必定

【导学】 necessity 所接的表语从句或同位语从句的谓语常用"（should）＋动词原形"，表虚拟语气。

【例句】 Is it a logical necessity that the cost of living will go up if wages go up?

【译文】 如果工资提高生活费用就要上涨，这是逻辑的必然吗？

negative ['negətiv]　　*a.* 否定的，消极的，反面的；负的，阴性的

【联想】 反义词 positive *a.* 正面的，积极的

【例句】 However, many studies of children's use of computers show that there are possible negative effects.

【译文】 然而，许多研究表明，儿童使用电脑可能存在负面影响。

neglect [ni'glekt]　　　　　　　*vt*. 忽视，忽略；疏忽

【例句】No country can afford to neglect education.

【译文】任何国家都不能忽视教育。

negotiate [ni'gəuʃieit]　　　　*v*. 谈判，交涉，商议

【搭配】negotiate with sb. about/over/on/for sth. 与某人谈判某事

【联想】negotiation *n*. 谈判

【例句】A veteran negotiation specialist should be skillful at manipulating touchy situations.

【译文】资深谈判专家应该善于处理棘手的局面。

negotiable [ni'gəuʃiəbl]　　　　　*a*. 可谈判的，可协商的，可通行的

neighbo(u)rhood ['neibəhud] *n*. 邻近，附近，周围

【搭配】in the neighborhood of 在……附近，大约

neural ['njuərəl]　　　　　　　*a*. 神经的，神经系统的

【例句】Obese women were nearly twice as likely to have a baby with neural tube defects.

【译文】妈妈肥胖，婴儿患神经管畸形（neural tube defects）的概率高达两倍。

neutral ['nju:trəl]　　　　　　　*a*. 中立的，中性的

【例句】She is neutral in this argument. She does not

care who wins.

【译文】 在这场辩论中她保持中立，不在乎谁赢谁输。

normally [ˈnɔːməli]　　　　　　　　*ad.* 一般；通常

【例句】 If your lively pets become passive, they might be ill normally.

【译文】 如果你活泼好动的宠物变得怠惰，通常可能是它们病了。

notwithstanding [ˌnɔtwiθˈstændiŋ] *prep.* 虽然，尽管
　　　　　　　　　ad. 尽管，还是 *conj.* 虽然，尽管

【例句】 You are what you eat notwithstanding, it is only recently that most consumers have become interested in the technical details of their food's composition.

【译文】 尽管饮食决定健康，但只是从最近开始大多数消费者才对他们所吃食物组成的技术细节感兴趣。

nuclear [ˈnuːkliə]　　　　*a.* 原子核的；核的，核心的

【例句】 Some scientists favor pushing asteroids off course with nuclear weapons.

【译文】 一些科学家更倾向于用核武器将行星从它们的轨道推出去。

nutrition [njuːˈtriʃən]　　　　　　　*n.* 营养，营养学

【联想】 nutritional *a.* 营养的

Day 17

machinery [məˈʃiːnəri]　　　　n. 机器；机关，结构

【导学】machine 是可数名词，表示机器；machinery 是不可数名词，表示机器的总称。

magic [ˈmædʒik]　　　　n. 魔法，巫术；戏法

magnet [ˈmægnit]　　　　n. 磁铁，磁石，磁体

magnetic [mægˈnetik]　　　　a. 磁的，有吸引力的

【例句】In order to be a successful diplomat you must be enthusiastic and magnetic.

【译文】想要成为一名成功的外交官，你必须热情且有魅力。

magnetism [ˈmægnitizəm]　　　　n. 磁，磁力，磁学

magnitude [ˈmægnitjuːd]　　n. 巨大，重大；大小，数量

【联想】magnify v. 使……变大

【例句】The destruction an earthquake causes depends on its magnitude and duration, or the amount of shaking that occurs.

【译文】地震造成的破坏程度由震级和持续的时间或者

震动发生的次数决定。

maintain [men'tein]　　　　　*vt.* 维持；赡养；维修

【例句】 The leaders of the two countries are planning their summit meeting to maintain and develop good ties.

【译文】 为保持并发展友好关系，两国的领导正在策划一场峰会。

maintenance ['meintinəns]　　*n.* 维持，保持；维修

mainstream ['meinstri:m]　　　　　　　*n.* 主流

male [meil]　　　　　*a.* 男的；雄性的 *n.* 男性

【联想】 female *a.* 女的；雌性的

malpractice ['mæl'præktis]　　　　　*n.* 玩忽职守

management ['mænidʒmənt]　　*n.* 管理；经营，处理

mankind [mæn'kaind]　　　　　　　　*n.* 人类

manifest ['mænifest]　　*a.* 明显的，显然的，明了的
　　　　　　vt. 明显，表明，证明；使显现，使显露

【例句】 The fact of first-rate importance is the predominant role that custom plays in experience and in belief and the very great varieties it may manifest.

【译文】 头等重要的事实就是风俗在信念和经验中所起的重要作用以及它所表现的众多变化形态。

---

manner ['mænə]　　　　　　*n*. 方式；态度；礼貌

【搭配】 all manner of 各种各样的，形形色色的；in a manner of speaking 在某种意义上

【例句】 Manners on the roads are becoming horrible.

【译文】 大街上的行为正变得越来越可怕了。

---

manual ['mænjuəl]　　　　*a*. 用手的，手工的；体力的
　　　　　　　　　　　　　　　　　　　　n. 手册

【联想】 manually *ad*. 手工地

【例句】 The ship's generator broke down, and the pumps had to be operated manually instead of mechanically.

【译文】 这艘船的发电机坏了，抽水机不能再机械运作了，必须由手工来操作。

---

manufacture [ˌmænju'fæktʃə]　　*vt*. 制造，加工
　　　　　　　　　　　　　　　　　n. 制造（业）；产品

---

manufacturer [ˌmænju'fæktʃərə]　　　　*n*. 制造者，
　　　　　　　　　　　　　　　　　　　制造商；制造厂

【例句】 Manufacturers said from the start that their pills offered a short-term therapy for the obese，not for people looking to fit into a smaller bathing suit.

【译文】制造商们从一开始就表示，他们的药物是为肥胖人群提供一种短期疗法，而不是为那些想要穿小一号泳衣的人准备的。

manipulate [məˈnipjuleit]　　*vt.* 操纵，利用，操作，巧妙地处理

【例句】In this exercise，we'll look at how we can manipulate the columns and rows in a table.

【译文】在此练习中，我们将了解如何处理表中的列和行。

margin [ˈmɑːdʒin]　　　　*n.* 页边空余；边缘；利润

【联想】marginal *a.* 边缘的

【例句】You shouldn't have written in the margin since the book belongs to the library.

【译文】既然这本书是属于图书馆的，你就不应该在页边空白处写字。

marine [məˈriːn]　　　　*a.* 海的，海产的；航海的，船舶的，海运的

marvellous [ˈmɑːviləs]　　　*a.* 奇迹般的，惊人的，了不起的

【导学】辨析 marvellous，wonderful：marvellous 形

容非凡得令人难以置信的东西；wonderful 指因未曾见过或不寻常而令人惊奇。

mature [məˈtjuə]　　　　　*a.* 成熟的；考虑周到的
　　　　　　　　　　　　　　　v. (使) 成熟，长成

【联想】immature *a.* 不成熟的；maturity *n.* 成熟

【导学】辨析 mature, ripe：mature 用于人时，指生理和智力发展到了成年，用于物时，指机能发展到可以开花结果，还可指想法、意图等"经过深思熟虑的"；ripe 用于物时，指植物的果实完全成熟，可以食用，也可指时机"成熟的，适宜的"。

【例句】Boys mature more slowly than girls both physically and psychologically.

【译文】无论在生理上还是心理上，男孩都比女孩成熟得晚。

maximum [ˈmæksiməm]　　　　*n.* 最大量，最高值
　　　　　　　　　　　　　　　　a. 最大的，最高的

【联想】minimum *n./a.* 最小 (量) (的)

【导学】maximum 的复数形式为 maxima 或 maximums。

【例句】The level of formaldehyde（甲醛）gas in her kitchen was twice the maximum allowed by federal standard for chemical workers.

【译文】在她家厨房，甲醛的浓度是联邦政府为化工厂的工人规定的最高标准的两倍。

means [miːnz]　　　　　　　　　*n*. 方法，手段，工具

【搭配】by all means 当然；by any means 无论如何；
by no means 决不；by means of 用，凭借

【联想】in any case，at any cost，one way or the
other 无论如何；under no circumstances，in
no respect，in no sense，in no way，on no
account，at no time 绝不

【例句】Though by no means rich，he was better off
than at any other period in his life.

【译文】尽管生活并不富裕，但他过得比以往任何时候
都好。

meantime ['miːn'taim]　　　　*n*. 暂时，期间
　　　　　　　　　　　　　　　ad. 同时，当时

measurement ['meʒəmənt]　　*n*. 测量，度量；
　　　　　　　　　　　　　　　尺寸，大小

【联想】measure *vt*. 测量

【例句】Combining the two measurements allows the
researchers to work out the distribution of fat
and water within.

【译文】结合这两种测量结果，研究人员可以计算出体
内脂肪和水分的分布。

mechanic [mi'kænik]　　　　　*n*. 技工，机械工人

mechanical [mi'kænikl]　　　*a.* 机械的；机械学的，
力学的；机械似的，呆板的

mechanism ['mekənizəm]　*n.* 机械装置；机构，结构
　　　　　　　　　　　　　　n. 奖章，勋章，纪念章

【例句】 It both probes the mechanisms involved in a
specific disease and suggests precise remedies.

【译文】 它既探讨了特定疾病的发病机制，又提出了精
确的治疗方法。

medium ['mi:djəm]　　　　*n.* 中间，适中；(*pl.* media)
媒体；媒介，媒介物；传导体 *a.* 中等的，适中的

【导学】 medium 的复数形式为 media。类似的词还有
datum—data。但应注意 premium—
premiums；gymnasium—gymnasiums。

【例句】 He is medium height.

【译文】 他是中等身材。

mediate ['mi:dieit]　　　　　　　　*v.* 仲裁，调停

【例句】 A better understanding of how caffeine medi-
ates these effects could help prevent these
health issues in people in the future.

【译文】 更好地理解咖啡因是如何介导这些效应的，有
助于预防未来人们出现这些健康问题。

medical ['medikl]　　*a.* 医学的；医疗；伤病的；
疾病的；内科的 *n.* 体格检查

【例句】Therapists cannot prescribe drugs as they are not necessarily medically qualified.

【译文】由于治疗师不一定具有行医资格，所以他们不可以开处方。

medication [ˌmediˈkeiʃn]　　　　　*n.* 药物

【例句】And anti-depressant medications may not be able to deal with all of those problems.

【译文】抗抑郁药物可能无法解决所有这些问题。

mental ['mentl]　*a.* 思想的；精神的；思考的；智力的；
精神病治疗的；精神健康的；疯狂的；发疯的
n. 精神病；精神病患者

mentality [menˈtæləti]　　　　*n.* 心态，思想方式

【例句】I cann't understand their mentality.

【译文】我理解不了他们的心态。

metabolism [meˈtæbəlizəm]　　　　*n.* 新陈代谢

【例句】Diabetes upsets the metabolism of sugar，fat and protein.

【译文】糖尿病扰乱了糖、脂肪和蛋白质的代谢。

methane ['miːθein]　　　　　*n.* 甲烷，沼气

migrate [mai'greit]　　　　　　v. 迁移，迁居；定期移栖

【联想】migrant n. 移居者；候鸟

【例句】We find that some birds migrate twice a year between hot and cold countries.

【译文】我们发现，有些鸟每年在热带与寒带国家之间迁徙两次。

millimeter ['milimi:tə(r)]　　　　　　n. 毫米

miniature ['minjətʃə]　　　　　　n. 缩图，缩影
　　　　　　　　　　　　　　　a. 微型的，缩小的

【例句】The toy maker produces a miniature copy of the space station, exactly in every detail.

【译文】这个玩具制造商制造了一种每个细节都很逼真的空间站缩微模型。

minimal ['miniməl]　　　　　　a. 最小的，最小限度的

minimum ['miniməm]　　　　　　n. 最小量，最低限度
　　　　　　　　　　　　　　　a. 最小的，最低的

【例句】It seems to be the minimum prerequisite.

【译文】忠诚是最起码的要求。

mislead [mis'li:d]　　　　　　vt. 使误入歧途；
　　　　　　　　　　　　　　　把……带错路；使误解

missile ['misail]　　　　　　　　*n*. 发射物；导弹

missing ['misiŋ]　　　　　　　*a*. 失去的，失踪的

【例句】John complained to the bookseller that there were several pages missing in the dictionary he bought.

【译文】约翰向书商抱怨说，他买的字典少了几页。

mission ['miʃən]　　　　　　　　*n*. 使命，任务

【搭配】on a...mission 负有……使命

misunderstand ['misʌndə'stænd] *vt*. 误解，误会，曲解

mitigate ['mitigeit]　　　　　　　*vt*. 减轻；缓和

【例句】It would help mitigate your discomfort.

【译文】这会帮你缓解不适。

moderate ['mɔdərit]　　*a*. 中等的，适度的；温和的，
　　　　　　　　　　　　　　　　　　稳健的

【例句】Her dietician suggested moderate exercise would help her recover soon.

【译文】她的营养师建议适度的运动可以帮助她很快康复。

moral ['mɔrəl]　　　　　*a*. 道德的，道义的，有道德的
　　　　　　　　　　　　　n. 寓意，教育意义

【联想】 morality n. 道德

【例句】 As regards the development of moral standards in the growing child, consistency is very important in parental teaching.

【译文】 对于成长中的孩子的道德水平的发展，一致性在家长的教导中是非常重要的。

motivate ['məutiveit] vt. 作为……的动机，促动；激励

【例句】 Examinations do not motivate a student to seek more knowledge.

【译文】 考试不能促使学生去追求更多的知识。

motive ['məutiv] n. 动机，目的 a. 发动的，运动的

mutation [mju:'teiʃn] n. 突变；（生物物种的）变异；（形式或结构的）转变；改变

【例句】 The virus mutates in the carrier's body.

【译文】 病毒在载体中发生变异。

mutant ['mju:tənt] a. 变异的，突变的

【例句】 The experts said the new vaccine can produce neutralizing antibodies for mutant COVID-19 strains found in Brazil.

【译文】 专家们说，这种新疫苗可以产生针对巴西发现的 COVID-19 突变株的中和抗体。

mutual [ˈmjuːtjuəl]   *a*. 相互的；共同的

【例句】He had taken the all-important first step to establish mutual trust.

【译文】为了建立相互信任关系，他迈出了最重要的第一步。

Day 18

vacant ['veikənt]   *a*. 空的；（职位）空缺的；茫然的

【联想】 vacancy *n*. 空缺

【例句】 Are there any rooms vacant in this hotel?

【译文】 这家旅馆有空房吗？

vaccine ['væksi:n]   *a*. 疫苗的，牛痘的 *n*. 疫苗

【联想】 vaccinate *v*. （给……）接种（疫苗）；（给……）打预防针

【例句】 Figures like these bring home the devastating impact of AIDS and the urgent need for a cheap, effective vaccine.

【译文】 这样的数据让人们了解了艾滋病毁灭性影响，人们急需一种廉价有效的疫苗。

vacuum ['vækjuəm]   *n*. 真空；真空吸尘器

【例句】 Her death left a vacuum in his life.

【译文】 她的去世给他的生活留下一片真空。

variable ['vɛəriəbl]   *a*. 易变的；可变的，可调节的 *n*. 变量

【例句】 Like any other system, it is highly variable.

【译文】和其他系统一样，这是高度可变的。

variation [ˌvɛəriˈeiʃən] *n.* 变化，变动；变种，变异

vary [ˈvɛəri] *vt.* 变化，改变

【搭配】vary with... 随……变化；vary from...to... 由……到……情况不同

【例句】The hopes, goals, fears and desires vary widely between men and women, between the rich and the poor.

【译文】无论男女，无论贫富，每个人的希望、目标、忧虑和愿望都大不相同。

vehicle [ˈviːikl] *n.* 车辆，交通工具

【例句】Cars and trucks are vehicles.

【译文】小汽车和大卡车都是交通工具。

venture [ˈventʃə] *n.* /*vi.* 冒险，拼，闯 *v.* 敢于，大胆表示 *n.* 冒险（事业）

【搭配】at a venture 胡乱地，随便地

【导学】辨析 venture, adventure, risk：venture 指冒生命危险或经济风险；adventure 指使人心振奋、寻求刺激性的冒险；risk 指不顾个人安危、主动承担风险的事。

verify [ˈverifai] *vt.* 证实，证明；查清，核实

【例句】 There are often discouraging predictions that have not been verified by actual events.

【译文】 经常会有未经事实证明的令人沮丧的预测。

veteran ['vetərən]　　　　　*n.* 老兵，老手 *a.* 老练的

via ['vaiə]　　　　　*prep.* 经，经由，通过

【例句】 I went to Pittsburgh via Philadelphia.

【译文】 我经过费城到匹兹堡。

vibrate [vai'breit]　　　　　*v.* (使) 振动，(使) 摇摆

【联想】 vibration *n.* 振动

【例句】 The diaphragm vibrates, thus setting the air around it in motion.

【译文】 膜片振动使得周围的空气也动荡起来。

violate ['vaiəleit]　　　　　*vt.* 违犯，违背，违例

【联想】 violation *n.* 违反

【搭配】 violate the regulation/agreement 违反规定/协约

【例句】 The actress violated the terms of her contract and was prosecuted by the producer.

【译文】 这位女演员违反了她合同的所有条款，因此被制片人起诉了。

virtual ['vəːtjuəl]　　　　　*a.* 虚的，虚拟的；实际上的

【联想】 virtually *ad*. 实际上

【例句】 Virtually，every cell in the body contains its own circadian clock machinery.

【译文】 实际上，身体中的每个细胞都有自己的生物钟。

virtue [ˈvə:tju:] *n*. 美德；优点

【搭配】 by/in virtue of 借助，经由

【例句】 The manager spoke highly of such virtues as loyalty，courage and truthfulness shown by his employees.

【译文】 经理高度评价员工所表现出的忠诚、勇气和诚实等美德。

virus [ˈvaiərəs] *n*. 病毒

【例句】 This is the pernicious virus of racism.

【译文】 这是种族主义的毒害。

vision [ˈviʒən] *n*. 视觉，视力；幻想，幻影；眼力，想象力；远见

【导学】 辨析 vision，sight，view：vision 指人的视力或视野，引申为远见卓识、美妙景色等；sight 指事物在人视线中的客观映象，引申为奇观、风景名胜等；view 指视线、视野时，可与 sight 互换使用，但 view 可指运用视力直接观察事物，也可指问题的角度、个人意见、美景等。

【例句】 Video game players may get an unexpected benefit from blowing away bad guys — better vision.

【译文】 电子游戏玩家可能会从赶走坏人中获得意想不到的好处——更好的视力。

visual ['viʒuəl]   *a*. 视觉的

【例句】 Playing "action" video games improves a visual ability crucial for tasks like reading and driving at night.

【译文】 玩"动作"游戏可以提高视觉能力,这对夜间阅读和驾驶等任务至关重要。

vital ['vaitl]   *a*. 极其重要的,致命的;生命的; 有生机的

【搭配】 be vital to 对……极其重要

【导学】 It's vital that 从句谓语动词用原形表示虚拟形式。

【例句】 The young people are the most active and vital force in society.

【译文】 年轻人是社会中最活跃、最有生气的力量。

vitamin ['vaitəmin]   *n*. 维生素

voluntary ['vɔləntri]   *a*. 自愿的 *n*. 志愿者

【例句】 There is a voluntary conveyance of property.

【译文】 这是一桩自愿的财产转让。

volunteer [ˌvɒlən'tiə(r)]　　　　　　*n*. 志愿者，志愿兵

【例句】 The team asked 6 healthy volunteers to wear electroencephalography（EEG）devices.

【译文】 研究小组要求6名健康志愿者佩戴脑电图仪。

vulnerable ['vʌlnərəb(ə)l]　　　　　　*a*. 易受攻击的，有弱点的；易受伤害的，脆弱的

【搭配】 vulnerable to 易受伤害的，易受打击的（其中 to 为介词，后面需接名词或名词短语）

【例句】 Some researchers feel that certain people have nervous systems particularly vulnerable to hot, dry winds. They are what we call weather-sensitive people.

【译文】 一些研究人员认为，有些人的神经系统特别容易受到干燥的热风的影响，他们就是我们所说的对天气敏感的人。

wisdom ['wizdəm] *n*. 智慧，明智；名言，格言；古训

withdraw [wið'drɔː]　　　　　　*vt*. 收回，撤回，提取
　　　　　　　　　　　　　　　　vi. 撤退，退出

【联想】 withdrawal *n*./*a*. 撤回（的）

【搭配】 withdraw...from... 将……从……撤回
　　　　 withdraw from 退出

【例句】 If after education he or she still shows no change，the Party branch shall persuade him or her to withdraw from the Party.

【译文】 经教育仍无转变的人，党支部应当劝其退党。

withstand [wið'stænd]　　　　　*vt.* 抵抗，经受住

【例句】 The new beach house on Sullivan's Island should be able to withstand a Category 3 hurricane with peak winds of 179 to 209 kilometers per hour.

【译文】 在沙利文岛的海边房屋应该能够抵挡 3 级飓风，这种飓风的最高风速为每小时 179～209 公里。

worthless ['wəːθlis]　　　　*a.* 无价值的，无用的

worthwhile ['wəːð'(h)wail]　　*a.* 值得（做）的

worthy ['wəːði]　*a.* 有价值的，可尊敬的；值……的，足以……的

【搭配】 be worthy of... 值得……的

be worthy to do... 值得去做……

【联想】 it is worthwhile to do sth. /sth. is worth doing 值得做某事

【导学】 sth. is worth（doing）（接名词或动名词）

sth. is worthy to be done（接不定式）

sth. is worthy of（接 of 短语）

it is worthwhile to do sth.（接不定式做主语）

sth. is deserving of（接 of 短语）

wreck [rek]　　　　　　　*n.* 失事，遇难；沉船，残骸

　　　　　　　　　　　　vt.（船等）失事，遇难

【例句】 He escaped from the train wreck without injury.

【译文】 他在这次火车事故中没有受伤。

wrist [rist]　　　　　　　　　　*n.* 腕，腕关节

【联想】 ankle *n.* 踝，踝关节；pulse *n.* 脉搏；palm *n.* 手掌；finger *n.* 手指；toe *n.* 脚趾

X-ray ['eks'rei]　　　　　　　*n.* X 射线，X 光

yearly ['jəːli]　　　　　　　*a.* 每年的，一年一度的

yield [jiːld]　　　　　*vt.* 生产，出产；让步，屈服

　　　　　　　　　　vi. 屈服，服从 *n.* 产量，收获量

【搭配】 yield to 向……让步

　　　　increase the yield 增加产量

【联想】 submit *v.* 屈服；obey *v.* 服从；compromise *v.* 妥协；surrender *v.* 投降

【例句】 They were short of sticks to make frames for the climbing vines, without which the yield would be halved.

【译文】他们缺少搭葡萄架的杆儿，没有它们葡萄产量就会减少一半。

zone [zəun]　　　　　　　　　　*n*. 地带，区域

【例句】Which time zone is your city located in?

【译文】你们的城市位于哪个时区？

wealthy ['welθi]　　　*a*. 富裕的，富有的，富庶的

【例句】He made his country wealthy and powerful.

【译文】他使国家富强了。

whereas [(h)weər'æz]　*conj*. 鉴于；然而，但是；反之

【例句】In the U. S. , the Republican's doctrines were slightly liberal，whereas the Democrats'were hardly conservative.

【译文】在美国，共和党的学说偏自由，而民主党几乎不保守。

widespread ['waidspred]

　　　　　　　　a. 普遍的，分布/散布广的

【例句】SARS is not a widespread disease.

【译文】SARS 并不是一个广泛传播的疾病。

附录一

医博英语真题词汇词频统计表

本词汇表为近十年真题试卷中词频在 10 以上的单词，使用的统计软件为 Wordcount。统计时同词根的派生词、合成词均独立计算，比如 she 和 she's 计算成两个词，分别统计词频。本次统计不含 Direction 中出现单词，更为准确。

单词	频率	单词	频率
the	5111	be	578
to	2576	on	524
of	2427	with	477
and	1666	as	464
in	1595	have	454
is	1282	from	446
that	986	What	445
for	774	can	402
It	648	You	380
are	602	not	365

（续）

单词	频率	单词	频率
by	362	people	206
Their	361	How	189
They	357	who	184
more	353	were	183
but	347	health	181
I	341	one	173
at	335	There	173
he	308	so	167
about	297	had	167
or	288	most	166
We	277	some	166
was	272	new	163
this	270	She	162
an	247	no	159
which	242	if	157
will	230	all	154
do	222	when	150
than	217	patients	149
has	215	out	147
his	212	may	146

单词	频率	单词	频率
been	145	says	113
would	142	disease	112
our	141	according	112
your	139	cancer	111
could	138	These	107
does	138	work	107
many	137	Them	107
medical	136	following	106
because	132	my	106
Research	129	now	104
should	128	Children	103
it's	126	well	103
other	125	two	102
study	121	way	100
up	121	just	98
Take	121	Its	97
time	120	world	95
man	118	need	93
like	118	day	92
her	113	use	92

（续）

单词	频率	单词	频率
much	92	woman	81
passage	91	make	81
too	90	human	81
only	90	good	80
Scientists	90	even	80
years	89	Why	80
first	87	any	80
such	87	doctor	80
over	85	weight	78
into	85	help	77
long	85	better	76
also	84	did	76
sleep	84	university	76
care	84	researchers	74
between	84	less	74
brain	83	problem	74
those	83	effects	74
get	82	me	74
medicine	81	science	73
author	81	think	73

单词	频率	单词	频率
Don't	73	test	61
change	72	best	61
year	71	problems	61
very	71	different	61
found	71	still	61
see	70	being	60
before	69	food	60
where	69	said	59
then	68	three	59
after	66	high	57
system	65	genetic	57
patient	65	blood	57
last	65	Both	56
doctors	64	go	56
know	63	likely	55
students	63	life	55
development	62	women	54
say	62	important	54
cells	62	countries	54
us	62	going	53

（续）

单词	频率	单词	频率
American	53	telemedicine	48
used	52	risk	47
Dr	52	own	47
mean	52	I'm	47
made	52	against	47
might	52	Little	47
same	51	body	47
often	51	probably	47
energy	51	diseases	47
through	51	scientific	46
right	50	around	45
off	50	Liver	44
results	50	times	44
school	49	That's	44
percent	49	really	44
climate	49	find	43
information	49	parents	43
animals	49	vaccines	43
him	49	drugs	43
during	49	TRUE	43

单词	频率	单词	频率
paragraph	42	come	39
obesity	42	pain	39
effect	42	bad	39
got	42	learn	39
without	42	public	38
family	41	enough	38
humans	41	possible	38
physical	41	exercise	38
lot	41	flu	38
case	41	feel	38
treatment	41	cause	38
part	40	global	37
among	40	few	37
studies	39	anything	37
while	39	talk	37
already	39	yes	37
future	39	back	36
heart	39	taking	36
diabetes	39	almost	36
difficult	39	another	36

（续）

单词	频率	单词	频率
must	36	Eat	35
great	36	early	34
surgery	36	having	34
million	36	loss	34
home	36	usually	34
give	36	develop	34
become	36	want	34
number	36	education	34
known	36	cannot	33
age	36	needs	33
child	36	Whether	33
result	35	young	33
each	35	tell	33
however	35	serious	33
every	35	days	33
reason	35	questions	33
several	35	job	33
place	35	today	33
past	35	yet	32
eye	35	ways	32

单词	频率	单词	频率
vaccine	32	Lower	31
growing	32	example	31
based	32	developed	31
History	32	down	31
changes	32	Next	31
Lab	32	never	30
impact	32	rate	30
caffeine	31	Second	30
put	31	culture	30
old	31	using	30
can't	31	vaccination	30
type	31	Doing	30
Healthy	31	Mental	30
means	31	hard	30
computer	31	current	30
under	31	far	29
provide	31	idea	29
White	31	poor	29
effective	31	Look	29
drug	31	understand	29

（续）

单词	频率	单词	频率
experience	29	services	27
social	29	water	27
program	29	low	27
Group	29	big	27
here	29	things	27
actually	29	thinking	27
birth	29	technology	27
week	29	art	27
able	29	States	27
feeling	29	practice	27
diet	28	behavior	27
always	28	HIV	27
understanding	28	value	27
reduce	28	makes	27
environment	28	infection	27
others	28	pills	27
live	28	set	27
something	28	highly	27
virus	28	Immune	27
I've	28	suggest	27

单词	频率	单词	频率
market	27	sperm	26
stay	27	data	26
exposure	27	person	25
control	27	Face	25
developing	26	given	25
country	26	companies	25
clinical	26	doesn't	25
months	26	since	25
biological	26	college	25
Adults	26	animal	25
obese	26	end	25
fat	26	United	25
ago	26	Answer	25
expected	26	green	25
men	26	although	25
model	26	hospital	25
seems	26	growth	25
therapy	26	treated	25
phone	26	form	25
least	26	making	25

（续）

单词	频率	单词	频率
knowledge	24	rather	23
insulin	24	term	23
thing	24	quality	23
man's	24	cases	23
small	24	neurons	23
learning	24	Sometimes	23
real	24	started	23
emissions	24	Short	23
increase	24	later	23
called	24	safety	23
hours	24	negative	23
meat	24	products	23
report	24	question	23
taken	24	smoking	23
sleeping	24	recent	23
show	24	available	23
kids	24	cost	22
side	24	keep	22
team	24	reported	22
environmental	23	Higher	22

单词	频率	单词	频率
inferred	22	thought	21
population	22	stress	21
left	22	weeks	21
morning	22	published	21
mother	22	beginning	21
trying	22	prevent	21
evidence	22	sure	21
fact	22	level	21
levels	22	ability	21
findings	22	general	21
half	22	relationship	21
particular	22	stop	21
depression	22	turn	21
factors	22	whose	21
suggests	22	training	21
further	22	activity	21
skills	22	believe	21
pay	22	greater	21
start	22	increased	21
though	21	benefits	20

(续)

单词	频率	单词	频率
lung	20	four	20
death	20	including	20
Try	20	view	20
Americans	20	ask	20
Once	20	whole	20
avoid	20	Fever	20
large	20	done	20
community	20	building	20
news	20	eating	20
lack	20	diagnosis	20
issue	20	cell	20
issues	20	word	19
clear	20	Free	19
room	20	healthcare	19
John	20	physician	19
eyes	20	caused	19
sense	20	senior	19
tests	20	simply	19
function	20	brains	19
within	20	working	19

单词	频率	单词	频率
soon	19	role	18
process	19	middle	18
systems	19	longer	18
nothing	19	hormone	18
government	19	pressure	18
kind	19	potential	18
mobile	19	mainly	18
mind	19	illness	18
differences	19	Air	18
lead	19	roofs	18
necessary	19	theory	18
safe	19	seem	18
average	19	describe	18
common	19	certain	18
class	19	patient's	18
OK	19	drinks	18
What's	19	led	18
hour	19	success	18
schools	19	structure	18
lives	19	rats	18

（续）

单词	频率	单词	频率
project	18	title	17
away	18	attention	17
coffee	18	radiation	17
affect	18	antibiotics	17
giving	18	shows	17
natural	18	carbon	17
dangerous	18	else	17
open	18	getting	17
condition	18	families	17
month	18	catch	17
service	18	ten	17
until	18	again	17
donor	18	looking	17
product	18	alone	17
bit	18	specific	17
clinic	18	light	17
children's	18	subjects	17
access	18	hospitals	17
CO	17	treat	17
response	17	began	17

单词	频率	单词	频率
laboratory	17	particularly	17
games	17	penicillin	16
personal	17	lose	16
perhaps	17	Tourism	16
night	17	didn't	16
weather	17	fast	16
normal	17	areas	16
offer	17	money	16
mentioned	17	produce	16
ones	17	Non	16
easy	17	along	16
members	17	wrong	16
worry	17	conducted	16
vision	17	emotional	16
asked	17	especially	16
planet	17	business	16
chronic	17	sick	16
improve	17	cough	16
consumers	17	conditions	16
amount	17	machine	16

（续）

单词	频率	单词	频率
examination	16	citizens	16
woman's	16	link	16
nature	16	plan	16
scientist	16	follow	16
genes	16	cut	16
efforts	16	Chinese	16
hope	16	th	16
company	16	infected	16
increasing	16	modern	15
call	16	cognitive	15
International	16	ear	15
play	16	Management	15
severe	16	remote	15
Despite	16	journal	15
phones	16	isn't	15
words	16	workers	15
designed	16	olds	15
came	16	positive	15
I'll	16	gene	15
five	16	Center	15

单词	频率	单词	频率
jobs	15	ideas	15
itself	15	living	15
caregivers	15	showed	15
conversation	15	robots	15
action	15	smaller	15
recently	15	approach	15
anti	15	difference	14
stomach	15	tumors	14
drink	15	abuse	14
minutes	15	society	14
significant	15	indeed	14
European	15	supposed	14
course	15	hand	14
build	15	concerns	14
earlier	15	pill	14
tumor	15	move	14
nearly	15	period	14
claims	15	overweight	14
costs	15	comes	14
car	15	childhood	14

（续）

单词	频率	单词	频率
ill	14	Advances	14
self	14	reality	14
monitoring	14	influenza	14
da	14	eight	14
professor	14	takes	14
similar	14	baby	14
technologies	14	due	14
works	14	benefit	14
tend	14	became	14
beef	14	hold	14
online	14	finding	14
doctor's	14	helps	14
trouble	14	quite	14
consumption	14	Oh	14
easily	14	terms	14
remain	14	bacteria	14
Vault	14	rates	14
scale	14	ever	14
portals	14	creativity	14
rise	14	Institute	14

单词	频率	单词	频率
together	14	skin	13
physicians	14	Redux	13
Spanish	14	coming	13
warning	14	Instead	13
epidemic	14	antibodies	13
medication	14	warming	13
cancers	14	African	13
German	14	successful	13
focus	13	colleagues	13
involved	13	stem	13
cold	13	across	13
point	13	evolution	13
summer	13	Throughout	13
deal	13	stage	13
brought	13	various	13
single	13	late	13
daughter	13	measure	13
everything	13	thinks	13
order	13	discovered	13
genome	13	wife	13

(续)

单词	频率	单词	频率
shown	13	mice	13
present	13	total	13
fear	13	challenge	13
themselves	13	livers	13
additional	13	saw	13
journals	13	perspective	13
restriction	13	I'd	13
Smith	13	contact	13
strong	13	killed	13
address	13	records	13
importance	13	department	13
major	13	bed	13
century	13	decade	13
treatments	13	main	13
Vinci	13	arts	13
California	13	died	13
changing	13	outbreak	13
communication	13	full	13
related	13	specialist	13
improved	13	lost	13

单词	频率	单词	频率
Specialists	13	argues	12
labels	13	gave	12
spent	13	combination	12
office	13	quickly	12
won't	13	suffering	12
happen	13	rule	12
visual	12	search	12
generalists	12	She's	12
There's	12	UK	12
entire	12	practices	12
completely	12	creative	12
gain	12	Let	12
combined	12	respond	12
operation	12	twice	12
provided	12	adult	12
noise	12	heat	12
friends	12	ray	12
reasons	12	seemed	12
run	12	standards	12
compared	12	Experts	12

（续）

单词	频率	单词	频率
Pasteur	12	damage	12
Prevention	12	demand	12
Biology	12	check	12
author's	12	industry	12
subject	12	agree	12
violent	12	cure	12
lived	12	failure	12
Chinatown	12	dioxide	12
behind	12	unique	12
Internet	12	sparrows	12
Africa	12	traditional	12
China	12	matter	12
interest	12	contamination	12
calories	12	aware	12
popular	12	groups	12
begin	12	wait	12
staff	12	moment	12
danger	12	San	12
critical	12	causes	12
symptoms	12	parts	12

单词	频率	单词	频率
feet	12	hearing	12
milk	12	technical	12
War	12	patterns	11
promising	12	teach	11
pandemic	12	tendency	11
goes	12	places	11
dogs	12	Telehealth	11
analysis	12	ready	11
coli	12	bring	11
rich	12	suggested	11
reduced	12	stock	11
grant	12	resistance	11
disorder	12	appointment	11
above	12	cars	11
teaching	12	organizations	11
mechanism	12	technique	11
measures	12	party	11
measles	12	survey	11
student	12	surgical	11
born	12	reports	11

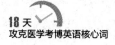

（续）

单词	频率	单词	频率
Talking	11	sort	11
anyone	11	worried	11
rabies	11	species	11
rapid	11	huge	11
buildings	11	extreme	11
prenatal	11	Wainwright	11
reach	11	faculty	11
phen	11	foods	11
range	11	ulcer	11
implies	11	Sleepwalking	11
spread	11	lifestyle	11
fall	11	Western	11
south	11	line	11
electronic	11	frequently	11
hundreds	11	local	11
method	11	game	11
statements	11	looked	11
involves	11	either	11
smallpox	11	greenhouse	11
meals	11	Finally	11
America	11	AIDS	11

单词	频率	单词	频率
Vegetative	11	name	11
COPD	11	thanks	11
fen	11	walk	11
math	11	Discipline	11
smiles	11	infections	11
account	11	Mr	11
goal	11	music	11
Henry	11	individual	10
injury	11	front	10
exposed	11	dream	10
He's	11	indicate	10
antibiotic	11	stroke	10
influence	11	tablets	10
writing	11	crucial	10
shape	11	chemical	10
heavy	11	seek	10
established	11	Freud	10
ward	11	phenomenon	10
National	11	remains	10
situation	11	Insomnia	10
You've	11	susceptible	10

（续）

单词	频率	单词	频率
drive	10	seen	10
grade	10	choose	10
serve	10	Germany	10
spend	10	Hitler	10
wealth	10	surgeons	10
dangers	10	extra	10
investment	10	widely	10
support	10	antiretroviral	10
universities	10	house	10
production	10	Ms	10
Protection	10	homes	10
pigs	10	explain	10
Policy	10	confirmed	10
Red	10	Conference	10
defects	10	temperature	10
break	10	took	10
Wednesday	10	near	10
source	10	parental	10
Arctic	10	received	10
psychologist	10	rules	10
crash	10	nice	10
generalist	10	nor	10

单词	频率	单词	频率
artists	10	whatever	10
babies	10	changed	10
association	10	stand	10
black	10	determine	10
they're	10	beneficial	10
risks	10	immigrant	10
testing	10	habits	10
English	10	feedback	10
reading	10	constant	10
gym	10	academic	10
maintain	10	wonder	10
exposome	10	diarrhea	10
economic	10	federal	10
Leukemia	10	felt	10
stopped	10	cord	10
caloric	10	economy	10
tried	10	manage	10
special	10		

注：由于篇幅所限，无法罗列全文。
请根据封面指示扫码获取词频统计表全文电子版。

附录二

小词大用

从附录一的词频表中可看出，真题中超高频率的单词往往是我们耳熟能详的虚词，比如冠词 the，a；介词 in，on，at；代词 this，that；连词 and，but。这些虚词往往一词多性，一词多义，除了在英语句子中充当极为重要的结构要素，还是完形填空、阅读理解以及翻译的考点。因此，在本部分，我们按照虚词的词性，结合词频，将这些小词分类别展示，并配套视频课程讲解。为节省篇幅，一词多性的小词只列入其中一类词性中讲解。

介词	*(prep.)*

aboard　　*prep./ad.* 在船（车、飞行器）上，上船（车、飞行器）

about　　*prep.* 关于，对于；在……周围，在……附近 *ad.* 在周围，附近；大约，差不多

　　联想　be about to（do）即将（不跟表示将来的时间状语连用）

above　　*prep.* 在……上面，超过 *a.* 上面的，上述的 *ad.* 在上面，以上

联想	above all 首先；尤其
	according to（表示依据）根据，按照
	across *prep.*/*ad.* 横越，横断
	prep. 在……对面
	after *prep.*/*conj.* 在……之后
	ad. 以后，后来
联想	after all 毕竟，终究；after a while 过了一会儿；be after 探求，寻找
against	*prep.* 对（着），逆；反对，违反；靠，靠近；和……对比
along	*prep.* 沿着 *ad.* 向前
联想	all along 始终，一直；along with 与……在一起；get along with 与……相处
among(st)	*prep.* 在……之中，在……之间
as	*prep.* 作为，当作 *conj.* 在/当……的时候；如……一样；由于，因为
联想	as... as 与……一样；as for/to 至于，就……而言；as if/though 好像，仿佛；as long as＝so long as 只要，如果，既然；as a matter of fact 事实上；as a result 结果；as far as... be concerned 就……而言；as follows 如下；as usual 照常
at	*prep.* 在……时，在……中；在……方面；向，朝；（表示速度、价格等）以

| before | *prep*. 在……前面 *conj*. 在……之前 |
| | *ad*. 从前，早些时候 |

联想 before long 不久以后；
long before 在……很早以前

| behind | *prep*. 在……后面，落后于 *ad*. 在后面， |
| | 落后 |

联想 fall behind = lag behind 落后；leave behind
留下；behind the times 落后于时代

| below | *prep*. 在……下面，在……以下 |
| | *ad*. 在下面；零度以下；下级 |

| besides | *prep*. 除……之外 *ad*. 而且，还有 |

| between | *prep*. 在……中间，在……之间 |
| | *ad*. 当中，中间 |

by	*prep*. 在……旁，靠近；被，由；在……
	前，到……为止；经，沿，通过；按照，
	根据 *ad*. 经过；（表示保留或保存时用）

联想 by hand 用手；by heart 牢记，凭记忆；
by oneself 单独地，独自地

| down | *prep*.（从高处）向下，顺……而下 |
| | *ad*.（坐，倒，躺）下，向下；下降；往南 |

| during | *prep*. 在……期间，在……时候 |

for	*prep*. 就……而言，对于；代，替，代表；
	（表示对象、愿望、爱好、活动等）为，为
	了，对于，给；（表示时间、数量、距离）

达，计；（表示目的、方向）向，对；（表示等值关系）换；（表示身份）当作，作为；（表示赞成、支持）拥护

联想 for all 尽管，虽然

from	*prep.* 从……起，从……来；出自；由于，因为；离；从，由
in	*prep.* 在（某范围或空间内的）某一点；（表示地点、场所）在……内
inside	*prep.* 在（或向）……里，在（或向）……内 *a.* 内部的，里面的；内幕的 *ad.* 在内部，在里面 *n.* 内部，里面，内侧
into	*prep.* 进入，到……里，成为，转为；（表示位置）在……里，在……中；（表示时间）在……期间，在……以后；（表示工具、方式）以……方式；（表示状态、情况）在……中，处于；（表示范围、领域、方向）在……之内，在……方面 *ad.* 向里，向内；在家里，屋里

联想 be in for 一定会遇到（麻烦等）；参加（竞争等）；in that 因为，原因在于

| like | *prep.* 像，和……一样 *a.* 相像的，相同的 *v.* 喜欢；希望；想要 |
| near | *prep.* 在……近旁，接近 *ad.* 接近，靠近；大约，差不多 *a.* 近，接近 *v.* 接近 |

附录二

265

联想 be near to 离……近的

of　　　　 *prep*.（表示从属关系）属于……的；由……
制成（或组成）的；含有……的，装有……
的；（表示性质、状况）；（表示位置，距
离）；关于；（表示同位关系）；（表示数量、
种类）；（表示部分或全部）；由于，因为；
（表示分离、除去、剥夺）；（表示行为主体
或对象）

off　　　　 *prep*.从……离开，离，偏离 *ad*.离，距，
离开，切断，停止，中止；完，光；剪
掉，扣掉；消除

联想 be well off 富有的；off and on 断断续续
地，间歇地，有时

on　　　　 *prep*.在……上；靠近，在……旁；关于，
有关；在……时候，在……后立即；朝，
向；针对；凭，根据；向前，（继续）下
去；在从事……中，处于……情况；在……
供职，（是）……成员 *ad*.（放、穿、连
接）上；向前，（继续）下去

联想 and so on 等等；off and on 断断续续地，
不时地；on and on 不断地

onto　　　 *prep*.到……上

outside　　 *prep*.在……外 *n*./*a*.外面（的），外表
（的），外界（的）*ad*.在外面，向外面

over	*prep.* 在……上方；高于，超过；在（做）……时候；越过，横跨；关于，在……方面；到处，遍及 *ad.* 翻过来；以上，超过；越过；再，又 *a.* 上面的，结束的
	联想 all over again 再一次，重新；over and over（again）一再地，再三地；over and above 另外，此外
past	*prep.* 过，经过 *a.* 过去的 *n.* 过去，昔日，往事
plus	*prep.* 加 *a.* 正的，加的 *n.* 加号，正号
round	*prep.* 围绕 *a.* 圆的，球形的；往返的 *ad.* 在周围 *v.* 绕行，使成圆形 *n.* 一圈，一周；巡回
	联想 all round 周围，处处；get round to do sth. = get round doing sth.（处理完其他事情后）终于能做某事
since	*prep.* 自从，从……以来 *conj.* 自从，从……以来；因为，既然 *ad.* 从那以后
through	*prep.* 通过，穿过；因为，由于；自始至终 *ad.* 通过，穿过；自始至终；彻底地，完全地；（打电话）接通
	联想 be through with 已结束
throughout	*prep.* 遍及，贯穿 *ad.* 到处，自如自终

附录二

till	*prep. / conj.* 直到……为止，直到
	联想 it is not untill... that 直到……才
to	*prep.* 向，往，至；对于；比，对；（程度、范围）过；到，（时间）在……之前，直到……为止
toward(s)	*prep.*（表示运动方向）朝，向；（表示关系）对于；（表示时间）将近；（表示目的）为了
under	*prep.* 在……下面；少于，低于；在……指导下；在……情况下；在……中
	联想 under way 进行中
unlike	*prep.* 不像……，与……不同 *adj.* 不同的，不相似的
up	*ad.* 向上；向（北方）；起床，起来；完全，彻底地 *prep.* 向上，向/在高处；沿着，溯流而上 *a.* 向上的
upon	*prep.* 在……上；朝向，向着 *ad.* 向前，继续
until	*prep.* 直到……为止，在……以前，直到……
with	*prep.* 和……一起；用；具有，带有；关于，就……而言；因为，由于；随着；虽然，尽管
within	*prep.* 在……里面，在……以内
without	*prep.* 毫无，没有 *ad.* 没有，缺乏
	联想 do without 没有……也行，不需要

代词　　　　　　　　　　　　　　　　　　　（*pron.*）

any	*pron.*无论哪个，无论哪些，任一，任何一些 *det.*任何的，任一的
anybody	*pron.*某人，随便哪一个人，无论谁，任何人
anyone	*pron.*某人，随便哪一个人，无论谁，任何人
anything	*pron.*任何事，任何东西（用于否定、疑问、条件句中），无论什么东西（事情）
anywhere	*pron.*无论哪里；（用于否定、疑问、条件句中）任何地方
both	*pron.*，*det.*两个，两个都
each	*pron.*/*det.*每个，各，各自
联想	each other 互相
either	*pron.*（两者中的）任何一个 *adv.*也（不），（补充时说）而且 *conj.*两者都（不），或者，要么
everybody	*pron.*每人，人人，各人
everyone	*pron.*每人，人人，各人
everything	*pron.*一切，每件事，凡事
most	*pron.*最大量，大多数，大部分 *det.*最多的，最大程度的，大部分的 *ad.*最，最大，非常

much	*pron.*许多，大量 *det.*许多的 *ad.*很，非常；……得很多，更……；几乎，大概
neither	*pron.*两者都不 *det.*（两者）都不的 *ad.*（否定的陈述同样适用其他人或物）也不；（否定的陈述适用于两方面）既不……也不…… *conj.*即不；也不
nobody	*pron.*没有人，没有任何人 *n.*小人物；无足轻重的人
none	*pron.*没有一个，无一 *ad.*一点都不
nothing	*pron.*什么也没有 *n.*微不足道的人或事
one	*pron.*一个人，任何人 *num.*一，一个 *det.*一个的，某一……的，同一的
other	*pron.*其他的人或事 *det.*其他的，别的
own	*pron./a.*自己的 *vt.*拥有
same	*pron.*同样的人或事 *a.*相同的，一样的
some	*pron.*几个，有些人 *det.*一些，少许，有些，某个，大约 *ad.*大约，稍微
somebody	*pron.*有人，某人
someone	*pron.*某人，有人
something	*pron.*某事，某物，（表示不确切的描述或数量）大致，在右
that	*pron.*那，那个；（引导定语从句）*conj.*（引导名词从句）*ad.*那样，那么

these	*pron.*（this 的复数）这些
this	*pron.*这，这个
those	*pron.*（that 的复数）那些
what	*pron.*什么，什么东西 *det.*多么；什么；……的事物
whatever	*pron.*无论什么，任何……的事物 *det.*不管怎么样的，无论什么样的
where	*pron.*什么地方 *ad.*在哪里；在……地方 *conj.*在……的地方
which	*pron.*哪一个，哪一些；（明确所指的事物）……的那个，那些 *det.*哪一个，哪一些
whichever	*pron./a.*无论哪个，无论哪些
who	*pron.*谁，什么人；……的人；（进一步提供有关某人的信息）
whoever	*pron.*谁，无论谁，不管谁，究竟是谁
whom	*pron.*谁
whose	*pron.*谁的，哪个（人）的，哪些（人）的

连词　　　　　　　　　　　　　　　　　　　　（*conj.*）

although	*conj.*尽管；虽然
and	*conj.*和，与，及；那么，则
联想	both... and 既……又；and so forth 等等；and so on 等等

because	*conj.* 因为
联想	because of 由于，因为；due to = owing to 由于，因为；thanks to 由于，幸亏
before	*conj.* 在……之前 *prep.* 在……前面 *ad.* 从前，早些时候
联想	before long 不久以后；long before 在……很早以前
however	*conj.* 然而，可是，不过 *ad.* 不管怎样
if	*conj.* 如果，假如；是否
nor	*conj.* 也不
now	*conj.* 既然 *ad.* 现在，目前，立刻 *n.* 现在，此刻
or	*conj.* 或，或者；即；否则，要不然
联想	or else 否则；or so 大约；or rather 或者更确切地说
otherwise	*conj.* 否则，要不然 *ad.* 另外，别样
so	*conj.* 因而，所以，结果是；为的是，以便 *ad.* 那么，如此；非常，很；也同样
than	*conj.* 比
though	*conj.* 尽管，虽然 *ad.* 可是，然而，不过
unless	*conj.* 如果不，除非
whenever	*conj.* 无论何时，随时，每当
wherever	*conj.* 无论在（到）哪里 *ad.* 究竟在

（到）哪里

whether   *conj.* 是否；不管，无论

while   *conj.* 当……的时候，和……同时；然而，虽然，尽管 *n.* 一会儿，（一段）时间

yet   *conj.* 然而，不过 *ad.* 到目前为止；更；还；总有一天仍然